Clinical Cases in
Gerodontology

Clinical Cases Series

Wiley-Blackwell's Clinical Cases series is designed to recognize the centrality of clinical cases to the dental profession by providing actual cases with an academic backbone. This unique approach supports the new trend in case-based and problem-based learning. Highly illustrated in full color, the Clinical Cases series utilizes a format that fosters independent learning and prepares the reader for case-based examinations.

Clinical Cases in Pediatric Dentistry (2nd edition)
by Amr M. Moursi (Editor) and Amy L. Truesdale (Associate Editor)
December 2019

Clinical Cases in Dental Hygiene
by Cheryl M. Westphal Theile, Mea A. Weinberg, and Stuart L. Segelnick
January 2019

Clinical Cases in Endodontics
by Takashi Komabayashi
November 2017

Clinical Cases in Orofacial Pain
by Malin Ernberg, Per Alstergren
March 2017

Clinical Cases in Implant Dentistry
by Nadeem Karimbux (Editor), Hans-Peter Weber (Editor)
December 2016

Clinical Cases in Orthodontics
by Martyn T. Cobourne, Padhraig S. Fleming, Andrew T. DiBiase, Sofia Ahmad
June 2012

Clinical Cases in Periodontics
by Nadeem Karimbux
December 2011

Clinical Cases in Prosthodontics
by Leila Jahangiri, Marjan Moghadam, Mijin Choi, Michael Ferguson
October 2010

Clinical Cases in Restorative and Reconstructive Dentistry
by Gregory J. Tarantola
September 2010

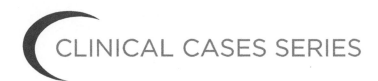

Clinical Cases in
Gerodontology

FIRST EDITION

Edited by

Gerry McKenna

BDS, MFDS RCSEd, PhD, FDS (Rest Dent) RCSEd, FHEA, FDTFEd
Clinical Reader and Consultant in Restorative Dentistry,
Centre for Public Health,
Queen's University Belfast,
United Kingdom

Finbarr Allen

BDS, MSc, PhD, FDS RCPS, FDS (Rest Dent) RCPS, FFD RCSI
Professor and Dean,
Faculty of Dentistry,
National University of Singapore,
Singapore

Francis Burke

BDentSc, MSc, PhD, FDS RCSEd, FFD RCSI, DipTLHE
Senior Lecturer and Consultant in Restorative Dentistry,
Deputy Head (Academic Affairs),
College of Medicine and Health,
University College Cork,
Ireland

WILEY Blackwell

Registered Offices
John Wiley & Sons, Inc., 111 River Street, Hoboken, NJ 07030, USA
John Wiley & Sons Ltd, The Atrium, Southern Gate, Chichester, West Sussex, PO19 8SQ, UK

Editorial Office
9600 Garsington Road, Oxford, OX4 2DQ, UK

For details of our global editorial offices, customer services, and more information about Wiley products visit us at www.wiley.com.

Wiley also publishes its books in a variety of electronic formats and by print-on-demand. Some content that appears in standard print versions of this book may not be available in other formats.

Library of Congress Cataloging-in-Publication Data

Names: McKenna, Gerry, 1980– editor. | Allen, P. Finbarr, editor. | Burke, Francis, 1959– editor.
Title: Clinical cases in gerodontology / [edited by] Gerry McKenna, Finbarr Allen, Francis Burke.
Other titles: Clinical cases (Ames, Iowa)
Description: First edition. | Hoboken, NJ : Wiley-Blackwell, 2021. | Series: Clinical cases series | Includes bibliographical references and index.
Identifiers: LCCN 2021007228 (print) | LCCN 2021007229 (ebook) | ISBN 9781119226598 (paperback) | ISBN 9781119226604 (adobe pdf) | ISBN 9781119226611 (epub)
Subjects: MESH: Dental Care for Aged | Geriatric Dentistry–methods | Case Reports
Classification: LCC RK55.A3 (print) | LCC RK55.A3 (ebook) | NLM WU 490 | DDC 618.97/76–dc23
LC record available at https://lccn.loc.gov/2021007228
LC ebook record available at https://lccn.loc.gov/2021007229

Cover Design: Wiley
Cover Images: © Courtesy of Gerry McKenna

Set in 10/13 pt Univers Light by SPi Global, Pondicherry, India
Printed and bound by CPI Group (UK) Ltd, Croydon, CR0 4YY

C063710_010321

CONTENTS

CONTENTS

Chapter 3   Management of Failing
Restorations   97

Chapter 4   Management of Malignancy and Other Oral Conditions   127

LIST OF CONTRIBUTORS

Editors

Finbarr Allen, National University of Singapore, Singapore

Francis Burke, University College Cork, Ireland

Gerry McKenna, Queen's University Belfast, United Kingdom

Contributors

Paul Brady, University College Cork, Ireland

Paul Brocklehurst, Bangor University, United Kingdom

Nico Creugers, Radboud University Nijmegen, the Netherlands

Cristiane da Mata, University College Cork, Ireland

Anneloes Gerritsen, Radboud University Nijmegen, the Netherlands

Harald Gjengedal, University of Bergen, Norway

Martina Hayes, University College Cork, Ireland

Nicola Holland, Belfast Health and Social Care Trust, United Kingdom

Christopher Irwin, Queen's University Belfast, United Kingdom

Simon Killough, Belfast Health and Social Care Trust, United Kingdom

Claudio Leles, Federal University of Goias, Brazil

Conor McLister, Belfast Health and Social Care Trust, United Kingdom

Haileigh McCarthy, Belfast Health and Social Care Trust, United Kingdom

Ciaran Moore, Queen's University Belfast, United Kingdom

Graham Quilligan, University College Cork, Ireland

Brian Rosenberg, BUPA Dental Care, Stalybridge, United Kingdom

Martin Schimmel, University of Bern, Switzerland

Murali Srinivasan, University of Zurich, Switzerland

Sayaka Tada, National University of Singapore, Singapore

Robert Thompson, Belfast Health and Social Care Trust, United Kingdom

Georgios Tsakos, University College London, United Kingdom

Celeste van Heumen, Radboud University Nijmegen, the Netherlands

Lewis Winning, Trinity College Dublin, Ireland

INTRODUCTION

With Contribution from Gerry McKenna, Finbarr Allen, Francis Burke, Paul Brocklehurst and Georgios Tsakos

Epidemiology of the Ageing Population

The global population is ageing. As a result of falling birth rates and significant increases in life expectancy, the proportion of older adults within the general population has increased markedly. This has been one of the most distinctive demographic trends of the last century and is predicted to continue at an increased rate into the next.[1] With fertility rates continuing towards lower levels, falling death rates become increasingly important in population ageing. In many more economically developed countries, where low birth rates have existed for a significant period of time, increases in the older population are now primarily as a result of improved chances of surviving into old age.[2,3] Over the next 50 years, global life expectancy at birth is projected to increase by 10 years on average, to reach 76 years in 2045–2050.[1] The gaps in life expectancy among more and less economically developed countries are predicted to decrease. Life expectancy at birth is expected to reach an average of 80 years in more economically developed countries, compared to 71 years in less economically developed countries.[1]

The generalised shift in the age distribution of mortality towards older groups means that more people will now survive into their seventh, eighth and ninth decades. Estimates suggest that almost three of every four newborns worldwide will now survive to 60 years, with one in every three living over 80 years. Not only are more people surviving to old age, but once there, they are living longer. Over the next 50 years global life expectancy at age 60 is expected to increase from 18.8 years in 2000–2005 to 22.2 years in 2045–2050 (an 18% gain), from 15.3 to 18.2 years (a 19% gain) at age 65 and from 7.2 to 8.8 years (a 22% gain) at age 80. These figures show that in fact the older the age group, the more remarkable are the expected relative gains in life expectancy.[1]

While the underlying reasons for improvements in life expectancy can differ depending on the country or region, common themes include increasing prosperity, education, public hygiene, improvements to housing and social welfare policies. Advances in healthcare provision have also played a pivotal role, including progression in preventative medicine, drug therapies and diagnostic tools. Unfortunately these advances have all come at increased economic costs for patients, healthcare providers or both.[4,5] In the United Kingdom, the Royal Commission on Long Term Care has estimated that the costs of caring for the elderly will quadruple in real terms between 1995 and 2051, from £11.1 billion to £45.3 billion.[6]

Due to the nature of chronic systemic conditions, the prevalence of these diseases is very high, with significant levels of co-morbidity reported among older patients.[7] They include cardiovascular disease, cancer, respiratory diseases and diabetes mellitus. Such chronic conditions are the leading cause of mortality worldwide and currently account for 63% of all deaths.[8] With life expectancy predicted to continue increasing, the burden of chronic illnesses among the older population will inevitably pose substantial medical, logistical and financial issues in the future.

The oral health of older adults

Older patients also suffer from chronic destructive oral diseases: dental caries and periodontal disease as well as toothwear. Caries and periodontal disease share many common risk factors with chronic systemic diseases, including smoking, poor-quality diet and a lack of glycaemic control. Although neither caries nor periodontal disease is a direct consequence of ageing, both are significantly more prevalent among older adults.[9] With increasing numbers of patients retaining natural teeth into old age, the burden of oral healthcare for the ageing population is also rising sharply, and since oral health conditions exert an excessive burden on older adults, oral health inequalities are therefore a major concern.[10]

The traditional picture of older patients with no natural teeth and complete replacement dentures is changing. Recent years have seen considerable improvements in the oral health of older patients, with a large number of epidemiological dental surveys indicating that levels of tooth retention have increased significantly in this age group.[11] Unfortunately, the cumulative nature of the two main destructive dental diseases, caries and periodontal disease, dictates that ageing will continue to be a factor associated with natural tooth loss.

Despite the overall prevalence of total tooth loss falling sharply in recent years, patients are now becoming edentulous at an older age, when they are often less able to adapt to the limitations of complete dentures.[12] The attitudes of older patients to oral health have also changed markedly, as they take advantage of widely available sources of information and ultimately demand more from clinicians. Increasing numbers of older patients are unhappy with treatment plans simply centred around extractions and replacement of natural teeth, and expect conservative treatment approaches instead.[13,14] Evidence suggests that has been a generational shift in patient attitudes to oral healthcare, with research illustrating that patients born after World War II have very different attitudes to oral health compared with those born pre-war.[15,16]

While increasing tooth retention represents a significant improvement in the oral health of the older population, it also brings with it the emerging challenges of managing chronic dental diseases for a new cohort. Factors including reduced manual dexterity and xerostomia coupled with a cariogenic diet mean that chronic dental diseases can cause considerable pain and suffering among older patients and can impair oral function.[17] Dental caries, particularly on root surfaces, remains a challenge for this age group, with high levels found among old-age populations, especially those living within residential care.[18,19]

The importance of oral health for older adults: links between oral disease and systemic well-being

Retention or replacement of missing natural teeth is important for restoration of oral function, aesthetics and quality of life. However, there is an ever-increasing amount of evidence to suggest that teeth and oral health are also very important for systemic health and well-being.[20] While a number of oral and systemic diseases can be linked by a variety of common risk factors, there is also evidence to suggest that there could be interactions between inflammatory periodontal diseases and conditions such as atherosclerosis, diabetes mellitus and respiratory diseases.[21] It has been shown too that as natural teeth are lost, chewing function can be negatively affected. This can have significant negative knock-on effects on dietary choice and overall nutritional status.[22] In older patients in particular, diet plays a very important role in systemic disease prevention, with poor diets implicated in bowel disease, osteoporosis and cardiovascular disease.

Therefore, it is important from both oral well-being and systemic health perspectives that oral health is maintained for older adults, ideally providing them with a pain-free, natural and functional dentition for life. In order to help oral health clinicians achieve this, there is a need to develop and provide training focused on gerodontology at undergraduate and postgraduate levels, both as part of formal programmes and through continuing professional development (CPD) opportunities.[23] Such opportunities should extend to the entire dental team, since all members have a role to play maintaining and improving oral health for older people.[24]

References

1 United Nations Department of Economic and Social Affairs (2001). *World Population Ageing 1950–2050*. United Nations, New York.
2 Grundy, E. (1996). *Population Ageing in Europe*. Oxford University Press, New York.
3 National Research Council (2001). *Preparing for an Ageing World: The Case for Cross-National Research*. National Research Council, Washington, DC.
4 Priest JL, Engel-Nitz NM, Cook CL, Cantrell CR (2012). Quality of care, health care costs and utilization amongst Medicare part D enrollees with and without low-income subsidy. *Population Health Management* 15: 101–112.
5 Van der Werf E, Verstraete J, Lievens Y (2012). The cost of radiotherapy in a decade of technology evolution. *Radiotherapy and Oncology* 102: 148–153.
6 Royal Commission on Long Term Care (1999). *With Respect to Old Age: Long Term Care – Rights and Responsibilities*. Stationery Office, London.
7 Naughton C, Bennett K, Feely J. (2006) Prevalence of chronic disease in the elderly based on a national pharmacy claims database. *Age and Ageing* 35: 633–636.
8 World Health Organisation (2005). *Preventing Chronic Diseases: A Vital Investment*. World Health Organisation, New York.
9 Steele JG, Treasure ET, O'Sullivan I, et al. (2012). Adult Dental Health Survey 2009: transformations in British oral health 1968–2009. *British Dental Journal* 213: 523–527.

10 Gerritsen AE, Allen PF, Witter DJ, et al. (2010). Tooth loss and oral health-related quality of life: a systematic review and meta-analysis. *Health and Quality of Life Outcomes* 8: 126.

11 Stock C, Jurges H, Shen J, et al. (2016). A comparison of tooth retention and replacement across 15 countries in the over-50s. *Community Dentistry and Oral Epidemiology* 44: 223–231.

12 Jepson NJ, Thomason JM, Steele JG (1995). The influence of denture design on patient acceptance of partial dentures. *British Dental Journal* 178: 296–300.

13 Cronin M, Meaney S, Jepson NJ, Allen PF (2009). A qualitative study of trends in patient preferences for the management of the partially dentate state. *Gerodontology* 26: 137–142.

14 Allen PF (2010). Factors influencing the provision of removable partial dentures by dentists in Ireland. *Journal of the Irish Dental Association* 56: 224–229.

15 Pearce MS, Steele JG, Mason J, et al. (2004). Do circumstances in early life contribute to tooth retention in middle age? *Journal of Dental Research* 83: 562–566.

16 Pearce MS, Thomson WM, Walls AW, Steele JG (2009). Lifecourse socio-economic mobility and oral health in middle age. *Journal of Dental Research* 88: 938–941.

17 Steele JG, Sheiham A, Marcenes W, et al. (2001). Clinical and behavioural risk indicators for root caries in older people. *Gerodontology* 18: 95–101.

18 Petersen PE, Yamamoto T (2005). Improving the oral health of older people: the approach of the WHO Global Oral Health Programme. *Community Dentistry and Oral Epidemiology* 33: 81–92.

19 Karki AJ, Monaghan N, Morgan M (2015). Oral health status of older people living in care homes in Wales. *British Dental Journal* 219: 331–334.

20 Seymour RA (2010). Is oral health a risk for malignant disease? *Dental Update* 37: 279–283.

21 Ford PJ, Raphael SL, Cullinan MP, et al. (2010). Why should a doctor be interested in oral disease? *Expert Review of Cardiovascular Therapy* 8: 1483–1493.

22 Moynihan PJ (2007). The relationship between nutrition and systemic and oral well-being in older people. *Journal of the American Dental Association* 138: 493–497.

23 Kossioni A, McKenna G, Müller F, et al. (2017). Higher education in gerodontology in European universities. *BMC Oral Health* 17: 71.

24 Kossioni A, Hajto-Bryk J, Maggi S, et al. (2018). An expert opinion from the European College of Gerodontology and the European Geriatric Medicine Society: European policy recommendations on oral health in older adults. *Journal of the American Geriatrics Society* 66: 609–613.

Chapter 1

Management of Chronic Dental Disease

Clinical Cases in Gerodontology, First Edition. Edited by Gerry McKenna, Finbarr Allen, and Francis Burke.
© 2021 John Wiley & Sons Ltd. Published 2021 by John Wiley & Sons Ltd.

Case 1

Management of Root Caries

With Contribution from Martina Hayes, Cristiane da Mata, Finbarr Allen and Francis Burke

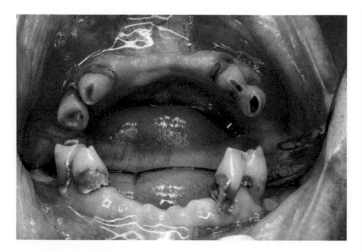

Figure 1.1.1 Circumferential root caries lesions affecting the remaining lower dentition.

A. Case Story

An 80-year-old female was admitted to a hospital ward following a stroke and a dental consultation was requested by her supervising medical team. She was wearing upper and lower acrylic partial dentures which had been constructed over 10 years ago. She had not attended her general dental practitioner since fabrication of the dentures as she had 'not had any pain from her teeth'. The woman was an inpatient in hospital and was medically frail. It was planned to admit her to a long-term residential care facility following discharge from the hospital as she would require a high level of nursing care, including feeding, toileting, bathing and dressing. A clinical examination revealed caries in her remaining natural teeth, particularly the partial denture abutment teeth (Figure 1.1.1). A clinical decision was made to manage the caries and to maintain the remaining natural dentition.

LEARNING GOALS AND OBJECTIVES

- Understand that root caries is a disease almost unique to older patients
- Understand the management of root caries and appreciate that restorations can have high failure rates
- Appreciate that glass ionomer cements, particularly high-viscosity glass ionomer cements, have been shown to have the highest success rates when restoring root caries lesions[1,2]
- Recognise that prevention or remineralisation of root caries must be implemented alongside any operative interventions

B. Medical History

- Previous stroke
- Patient very frail
- Rheumatoid arthritis
- Osteoporosis

C. Dental History

- Partially dentate and wearing upper and lower acrylic dentures constructed by her general dental practitioner approximately 10 years ago
- Patient has not attended a dentist for many years as her health has declined and she has found it difficult to travel

D. Medications

- Dabigatran (anticoagulant) 150 mg twice daily
- Clopidogrel (anticoagulant) 75 mg once daily
- Methotrexate (antimetabolite) 7.5 mg once weekly
- Ibuprofen (non-steroidal anti-inflammatory) 200 mg three times per day
- Alendronic acid (oral bisphosphonate) 10 mg once daily

E. Social History

- Widowed
- Patient was living independently until her stroke, due to enter long-term care facility after hospital discharge
- Non-smoker and does not consume alcohol

F. Extraoral Examination

- Medically frail
- Joints in fingers severely affected by rheumatoid arthritis

G. Soft Tissue Examination

- No significant findings

H. Clinical Findings/Problem List

- Partially dentate in upper and lower arch, patient wearing acrylic removable partial dentures; although worn, the dentures appear to be well tolerated and retained
- Oral hygiene poor, soft deposits present around all remaining natural teeth; no periodontal pocketing noted or mobility of remaining teeth

- Good oral lubrication, no evidence of xerostomia or salivary hypofunction
- Root caries evident in lower denture abutment teeth; no reported symptoms from carious teeth
- Evidence of toothwear on remaining upper dentition
- Tooth charting:

				4	3					4				
				4	3			2	3					

- Basic periodontal examination:

–	1	–
–	1	–

I. Diagnoses

- Chronic gingivitis
- Root caries
- Non-carious tooth surface loss
- Multiple edentulous spans

CLINICAL DECISION MAKING – DETERMINING FACTORS

- Patient has a very high caries risk and active root caries in her mouth. As a result of her recent stroke and rheumatoid arthritis, she has limited or no basic self-care ability. Following her stroke, this patient is now a high choking risk and her diet is soft or semi-liquid.
- In this case it is advisable to avoid extractions if possible, as the patient has been on bisphosphonate medication for a number of years and could be at risk of developing bisphosphonate-related osteonecrosis of the jaws (BRONJ).[3] In addition, the abutment teeth are helping to retain the patient's existing partial dentures.
- The patient will need oral care delivered at the bedside where possible as she is an inpatient in hospital. She is due to transfer to a residential facility where domiciliary visits will be required from a dental professional to help her maintain her dentition. Her carers will also require information on how to maintain her dentition.[4]
- It is very questionable if this patient has the ability to adapt to a new set of dentures. Although her existing dentures are worn, they are functional and reasonably well retained.

A discussion was had with the patient's family and her medical team regarding the provision of new partial dentures. The medical team explained that they did not envisage the patient progressing beyond a semi-liquid diet. Given the patient's frailty and the difficulty in fabricating a satisfactory set of prostheses, the decision was made not to begin making new dentures.
- The focus of any treatment now is to avoid any future dental problems that could cause pain and/ or infection.
- The treatment plan developed in this case included application of 22,600 ppm fluoride varnish every three months to reduce future caries risk and conservative management of carious teeth.
- The treatment was provided in a dental hospital with the patient transported via ambulance. The soft caries was excavated using a round bur in a slow-speed handpiece. Isolation was achieved using cotton-wool rolls and high-viscosity glass ionomer cement was placed (Fuji IX GP Extra™, GC Corporation, Japan). The restorations were covered with petroleum jelly to protect the glass ionomer cement during maturation (Figure 1.1.2).

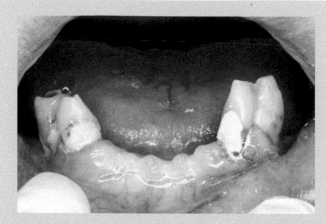

Figure 1.1.2 Glass ionomer cement (Fuji IX GP Extra™, GC Corporation, Japan) restorations placed on lower teeth.

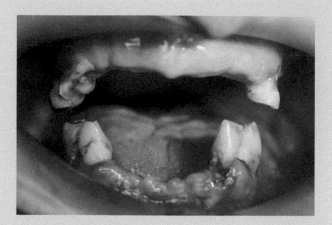

Figure 1.1.3 Patient at three-month review.

Restoration of root caries lesions is challenging as they exhibit mixed cavity margins positioned in enamel as well as dentine. The cavities also tend to be broad, shallow and saucer shaped, with no natural retention. Failure rates of root caries restorations can be as high as 68% at 1 year.[5] However, one study on high-viscosity glass ionomer cements achieved survival rates of 87% at 1 year.[6] Glass ionomer cements have also been associated with protection against secondary caries, even after loss of the restoration itself.

- High-fluoride varnish (Duraphat® 22,600 PPM Varnish, Colgate, USA) was applied to all the remaining natural teeth. This has been shown to reduce the incidence of new root caries lesions and is a non-invasive, low-risk, inexpensive treatment to provide in a professional or domiciliary setting.[7] However, the varnish should avoided in patients with stomatitis or those with asthma.

- The patient was seen again after three months for another application of fluoride varnish. At this appointment it was noted that the restoration in the 32 had been lost. The cavity was leathery to a ball-ended probe and it seemed likely that this lesion was inactive.[8] It was decided to keep this lesion under observation at the three-monthly fluoride varnish applications (Figure 1.1.3).

Self-Study Questions

1. Which population group is root caries most frequently detected in?
   a. Young adults
   b. Middle-aged adults
   c. Adults with heavily restored dentitions
   d. Older adults

2. Which material is most effective for restoration of root caries?
   a. Amalgam
   b. Composite resin
   c. High-viscosity glass ionomer cements
   d. Compomer

3. Which of the following are important aetiological factors in the development of root caries?
   a. Xerostomia
   b. Recurrent ulceration
   c. Denture stomatitis
   d. Angular cheilitis

4. What are the reasons that high-fluoride varnish application is recommended in the prevention of root caries?
   a. Expensive to deliver
   b. High risk
   c. Can be provided in a professional or domiciliary setting
   d. Little evidence to suggest effectiveness

5. Which of these matches the typical appearance of a root caries lesion?
   a. Broad, shallow and saucer shaped with no natural retention
   b. Well defined, arising at the contact point between adjacent teeth
   c. Deep, narrow lesions extending into the tooth
   d. There is no typical appearance

Answers are located at the end of the case

Self-Study Answers

1. d. Older adults[7]

2. c. High-viscosity glass ionomer cements[2]

3. a. Xerostomia[7]

4. c. Can be provided in a professional or domiciliary setting[1]

5. a. Broad, shallow and sauced shaped with no natural retention[7]

References

1 da Mata C, McKenna G, Anweigi L, et al. (2019). An RCT of atraumatic restorative treatment for older adults. *Journal of Dentistry* 83: 95–99.

2 Hayes M, Brady P, Burke FM, Allen PF (2016). Failure rates of class V restorations in the management of root caries in adults—a systematic review. *Gerodontology* 33: 299–307.

3 Scottish Dental Clinical Effectiveness Programme (2017). *Oral Health Management of Patients at Risk of Medication-related Osteonecrosis of the Jaw*. NHS Education for Scotland, Edinburgh.

4 Kossioni AE, Hajto-Bryk J, Janssens B, et al. (2018). Practical guidelines for physicians in promoting oral health in frail older adults. *Journal of American Medical Directors Association* 19: 1039–1046.

5 De Moor RJG, Stassen IG, van't Veldt Y, et al. (2011). Two-year clinical performance of glass ionomer and resin composite restorations in xerostomic head- and neck-irradiated cancer patients. *Clinical Oral Investigations* 15: 31–38.

6 Lo EC, Luo Y, Tan HP, et al. (2006). ART and conventional root restorations in elders after 12 months. *Journal of Dental Research* 85: 929–932.

7 Hayes M, Burke F, Allen PF (2017). Incidence and global distribution of root caries. *Monographs in Oral Science* 26: 1–8.

8 Hayes M, da Mata C, Cole M, et al. (2016). Risk indicators associated with root caries in independently living older adults. *Journal of Dentistry* 51: 8–14.

Case 2

Caries Management in a Long-Term Care Facility Using Atraumatic Restorative Treatment (ART)

With Contribution from Cristiane da Mata, Martina Hayes, Francis Burke and Finbarr Allen

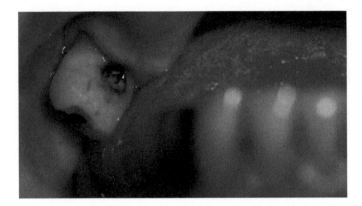

Figure 1.2.1 Carious lesion in an upper molar tooth.

A. Case Story

A clinical examination of a 76-year-old female patient in a long-term care facility revealed caries in a number of teeth (Figures 1.2.1 and 1.2.2). The patient reported no painful symptoms from her teeth. She did report that she felt her teeth were 'crumbling down' and found it difficult to brush and keep them clean. The patient wears an upper removable partial denture and has not received any dental treatment for a number of years. The long-term care facility does not have an active preventative oral care programme in place, but does contact local dental practitioners if residents report discomfort from their mouth or teeth. In this case management of caries was undertaken using atraumatic restorative treatment (ART) in a domiciliary setting.

LEARNING GOALS AND OBJECTIVES
- Be aware that a large proportion of residential care home residents still have some or all of their natural teeth
- Appreciate that provision of operative care in a domiciliary setting can be challenging and that pragmatic treatment planning decisions must be made

- Comprehend that the ART approach for caries management has been shown to be an acceptable and cost-effective strategy to treat carious lesions in the elderly, overcoming treatment barriers such as access, cost and patient acceptability.

B. Medical History
- Type II diabetes mellitus, well controlled with medication
- High blood pressure
- Atrial fibrillation
- Rheumatoid arthritis
- Osteoporosis
- Limited mobility

C. Dental History
- Patient has not attended a dentist for a number of years and has not received an oral examination since entering the residential care home

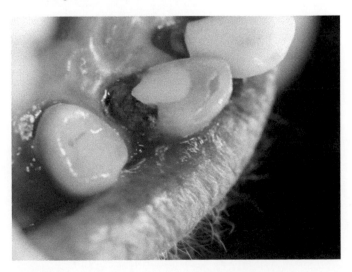

Figure 1.2.2 Carious lesion in an upper lateral incisor.

- Patient previously had multiple extractions in the upper arch due to caries and now wears an upper removable denture; she finds her upper denture comfortable
- Patient finds it difficult to brush and clean her teeth without assistance

D. Medications
- Clopidogrel (anticoagulant) 75 mg once daily
- Captopril (ACE inhibitor) 150 mg once daily
- Methotrexate (antimetabolite) 7.5 mg once weekly
- Alendronic acid (oral bisphosphonate) 10 mg once daily
- Diazepam (benzodiazepine) 10 mg once daily

E. Social History
- Widowed
- Retired nurse
- Patient living in a long-term care facility
- Non-smoker and does not consume alcohol

F. Extraoral Examination
- Patient is frail with limited mobility, able to sit in chair
- No other significant findings

G. Soft Tissue Examination
- No significant findings

H. Clinical Findings/Problem List
- Poor plaque control
- Areas of gingival recession and root restorations
- Active cavitated carious lesions in molar and anterior teeth
- Partially dentate in upper and lower arch, patient wearing upper acrylic removable partial dentures; patient has retained lower anterior teeth (shorted dental arch) and has never worn a lower prosthesis; patient has no functional or aesthetic deficit
- Mouth dry, evidence of xerostomia or salivary hypofunction
- Tooth charting:

		6				1	1	2	3	4			7	
				4	3	2	1	1	2	3			6	

- Basic periodontal examination:

–	1	1
–	2	–

I. Diagnoses
- Chronic gingivitis
- Coronal caries
- Root caries
- Missing teeth

CLINICAL DECISION MAKING – DETERMINING FACTORS

- Manual dexterity problems, loss of independence, lack of a prevention culture, xerostomia and the use of sugary medications often put patients in residential care homes at a high risk for dental caries.[1] As a result of a lifelong deposition of secondary dentine, they frequently do not present with pain until carious lesions become extensive and restorative treatment challenging.
- Treatment for patients in residential care homes often necessitates domiciliary care, as travel to dental surgeries can be extremely challenging and logistically difficult.[2]
- In order to prevent caries from occurring in these patients, or to diagnose lesions at their initial stages, making treatment less costly and simpler, the use of the minimal intervention dentistry (MID) approach is a useful tool, ultimately avoiding tooth loss and maintaining a functional dentition.

- MID is a concept born from the evolution in the understanding of the caries process and the mechanisms involved in its beginning, progression and control, together with improved dental materials. It consists of diagnosing and treating the disease caries as early and as minimally invasively as possible. It means prioritising prevention, patient information and guidance to empower them to be responsible for their own oral health and to intervene as conservatively as possible when a surgical approach is judged necessary, thus minimising tooth tissue loss. The aim of MID is to keep teeth healthy and functional for life and the strategies to achieve this by keeping teeth free from carious lesions include early caries detection and risk assessment; remineralisation of demineralised enamel and dentine; optimal caries preventative measures;

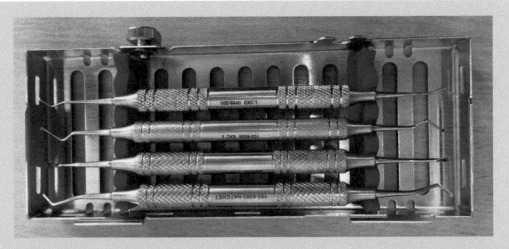

Figure 1.2.3 Basic atraumatic restorative technique instrument kit used for domiciliary care in this case.

minimally invasive operative interventions such as ART; and repair rather than replacement of restorations.[1]

- This patient has impaired manual dexterity and plaque control is poor. She also presents with active cavitated root lesions which are asymptomatic. They have a light brown colour, are covered with plaque, and carious dentine is easily scraped off with the use of a probe. The cavities are not self-cleansable and patient's oral health is poor, which could contribute to the progression of the disease process and size of the lesions. Therefore, restoration of the carious lesions at this stage using a minimally invasive approach such ART is indicated.[3,4]

- The treatment plan developed for this patient included extensive oral hygiene instruction provided for her carers including using of a high-fluoride toothpaste (Duraphat® 5000 ppm Fluoride Toothpaste, Colgate-Palmolive, UK) and denture cleaning instructions; restoration of carious lesions; and application of high-fluoride varnish (Duraphat® 22,600 PPM Varnish, Colgate, USA) at three-monthly intervals to all remaining natural teeth.

- Utilising the ART approach, caries was removed and restorations placed using hand instruments only (Figures 1.2.3 and 1.2.4). Enamel hatchets were used to create access to the caries lesions and excavators removed the very soft, demineralised dentine (infected dentine). Removal of tissue was stopped when some resistance on excavation was felt. The cavity was then washed with water spray and dried with cotton pellets.

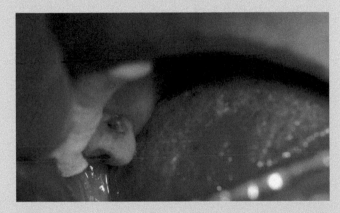

Figure 1.2.4 Cavity in upper molar after caries removal using hand instrument.

Moisture isolation was achieved with the use of a saliva ejector and cotton-wool rolls. A polyacrylic acid dentine conditioner (Dentin Conditioner, GC Corporation, Japan) was then used for 20 seconds. The acid was removed with a water spray and cotton pellets used again to dry the cavity but not desiccate it. A high-strength glass ionomer cement (Fuji IX GP Extra™, GC Corporation, Japan) was used to restore the cavity (Figures 1.2.5 and 1.2.6).

- Use of ART for restoration of carious lesions in older patients within a residential care setting produces survival rates which are similar to conventional rotary techniques.[5,6] The ART approach should be considered for providing dental care for older adults, particularly those in the non-clinical environment.

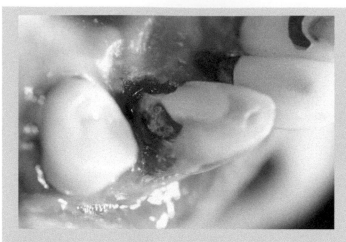

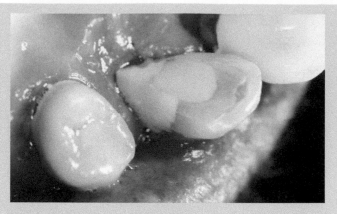

Figure 1.2.5 Cavity in upper canine after caries removal using hand instrument.

Figure 1.2.6 Glass ionomer cement (Fuji IX GP Extra™, GC Corporation, Japan) restoration placed on upper canine using ART approach.

Self-Study Questions

1. Atraumatic restorative treatment (ART) was first described as a clinical technique in which setting?
   a. Dental surgery
   b. Community dental clinic
   c. A non-clinical environment
   d. Dental hospital

2. Which of the following is an example of the concept of minimally invasive dentistry (MID)?
   a. Repair of existing restorations
   b. Provision of extensive crown and bridgework
   c. Non-surgical periodontal treatment
   d. Root canal treatment

3. Which instruments are used for removal of the carious lesion when applying the ART approach?
   a. High-speed rotary handpiece
   b. Slow-speed rotary handpiece
   c. Periodontal probe
   d. ART hand instruments

4. Which material is indicated for restoration of cavities prepared using the ART approach?
   a. Composite resin
   b. Amalgam
   c. Intermediate restorative material (IRM)
   d. High-viscosity glass ionomer cement

5. Which of the following chemical substances can be used to aid in the caries removal process during ART?
   a. Ozone
   b. Hydrochloric acid
   c. Carisolv
   d. Dentine bonding agent

Answers are located at the end of the case

Self-Study Answers

1. c. A non-clinical environment[3]

2. a. Repair of existing restorations[7]

3. d. ART hand instruments[3]

4. d. High-viscosity glass ionomer cement[5,6]

5. c. Carisolv[7]

References

1 Hayes M, da Mata C, McKenna G, et al. (2017). Evaluation of the cariogram for root caries prediction. *Journal of Dentistry* 62: 25–30.
2 Janssens B, Vanobbergen J, Petrovic M, et al. (2018). The impact of a preventative and curative oral healthcare program on the revalence and incidence of oral health problems in nursing home residents. *PLoS One* 13: e0198910,
3 Frencken JE, Peters MC, Manton DJ, et al. (2012). Minimal intervention dentistry for managing dental caries – a review. *International Dental Journal* 62: 223–243.
4 da Mata C, Allen PF, Cronin M, et al. (2014). Cost-effectiveness of ART restorations in elderly adults: a randomized clinical trial. *Community Dentistry and Oral Epidemiology* 42: 79–87.
5 da Mata C, Allen PF, McKenna G, et al. (2015). Two-year survival of ART restorations placed in elderly patients: a randomised controlled clinical trial. *Journal of Dentistry* 43: 405–411.
6 da Mata C, McKenna G, Anweigi L, et al. (2019). An RCT of atraumatic restorative treatment for older adults: 5 year results. *Journal of Dentistry* 83: 95–99.
7 Hayes M, Allen E, da Mata C, et al. (2014). Minimal intervention dentistry and older patients part 2: minimally invasive operative interventions. *Dental Update* 41: 500–505.

Case 3

Non-surgical Periodontal Treatment (NSPT) for Periodontally Involved Lower Incisors

With Contribution from Lewis Winning and Christopher Irwin

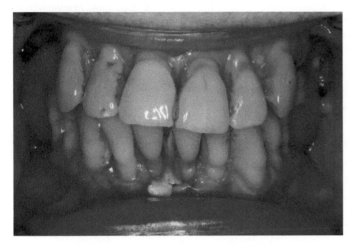

Figure 1.3.1 Clinical presentation of patient before treatment.

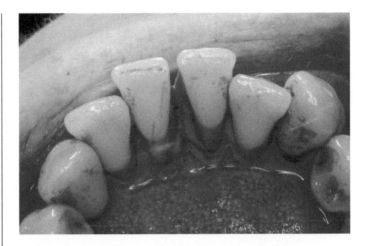

Figure 1.3.2 Calculus deposits on lower anterior teeth.

A. Case Story

A 72-year-old female presented complaining of receding gums, slight mobility of the lower incisors, and general concern for the prognosis of her remaining dentition. Clinical and radiographic examination revealed a diagnosis of generalised moderate chronic periodontitis with localised severe disease affecting the lower incisor teeth. The patient admitted that she struggled with maintenance of oral hygiene, particularly in the lower incisor region. Oral hygiene was poor throughout the mouth, with supragingival deposits clearly visible on the lower incisors (Figures 1.3.1 and 1.3.2). There was Grade I mobility of the lower right and lower left central incisors, with approximately 80% bone loss around these teeth (Figure 1.3.3).

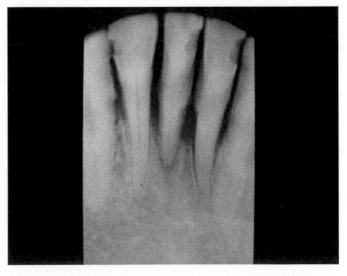

Figure 1.3.3 Radiographic findings at initial presentation.

LEARNING GOALS AND OBJECTIVES

- Understand that the prevalence and severity of periodontitis increase with age.[1] Previous interpretation of these data suggested that age itself could be a risk factor for periodontal disease.
- Recognise that ageing has been associated with a decline in immune responses, including mucosal immunoglobulin (Ig) M levels, cytokines and markers for B- and T-cells.[2,3]
- Understand that oral microbiological changes have also been proposed as a theory to explain the higher prevalence and/or severity of periodontitis in older adults.[4]
- Appreciate that due to the lack of direct evidence, the current view is that the greater level of periodontal destruction seen in older populations reflects more an accumulation of disease over a lifetime and not an age-specific condition.[5]

B. Medical History

- Mild osteoporosis
- Arthritis affecting the patient's hands
- Atrial fibrillation

C. Dental History

- Partially dentate but no experience of removable dentures
- Regular dental attender, but previously had not attended for a number of years
- Patient has previously lost posterior teeth due to periodontal disease
- Patient is aware that she suffers from periodontal disease

D. Medications

- Warfarin (anticoagulant) 2 mg daily
- Aspirin (non-steroidal anti-inflammatory) 150 mg daily
- Calcium carbonate (dietary supplement) 500 mg twice daily
- Propranolol hydrochloride (beta blocker) 80 mg twice per day
- Simvastatin (CoA reductase inhibitor) 40 mg once daily

E. Social History

- Retired, previously a part-time office worker
- Previous smoker, quit approximately 15 years ago
- Alcohol: less than 10 units per week

F. Extraoral Examination

- No significant findings

G. Soft Tissue Examination

- Gingivae around lower incisors inflamed
- No other significant findings

H. Clinical Findings/Problem List

- Partially dentate in upper and lower arches
- Oral hygiene poor, soft and hard deposits present
- Lower incisors grade I mobile
- Radiographic examination revealed approximately 70% horizontal bone loss associated with lower incisor teeth
- No denture-wearing experience
- Tooth charting:

	7			3	2	1	1	2	3		6	7	
8		5	4	3	2	1	1	2	3	4		7	

- Basic periodontal examination:

–	2	–
2	2	–

I. Diagnosis

- Chronic generalised periodontal disease
- Grade I mobile lower incisors

CLINICAL DECISION MAKING – DETERMINING FACTORS

- The decision whether to maintain or extract compromised dentition depends on a range of factors and is specific to the individual patient. With such advanced bone loss and the obvious difficulty in maintaining hygiene in this area, a good argument could be constructed for removal of both the lower right and lower left central incisors.
- However, this must be balanced by the fact this patient already has a reduced but functional dentition. Further tooth loss would likely necessitate a partial denture, which as discussed in other cases can have low acceptance rates and expedite further periodontal deterioration in the remaining dentition.[6]
- In this case, after discussion with the patient, a decision was made to maintain her current dentition. A treatment plan was drawn up including oral hygiene instruction, non-surgical periodontal therapy, review and regular maintenance therapy (Figures 1.3.4, 1.3.5 and 1.3.6).
- It was stressed to the patient that routine dental maintenance would be a key determining factor in tooth longevity. It has been shown previously that even teeth with advanced bone loss can be maintained as part of a functional dentition over long periods of time.[7] A further option would have been to splint the lower incisors; however, as the mobility was grade I and there was no functional interference, this was not indicated.
- Treatment was performed uneventfully and the patient adhered to a strict three-monthly maintenance regime with her dental hygienist, with annual periodontal review.
- Periodontal therapy in older patients must be adjusted to medical conditions, access to care, affordability and the ability to perform adequate oral hygiene.[8]
- Plaque control is central to the treatment of inflammatory periodontal disease. While self-performed plaque control is not in itself directly related to age, in the older patient it is much more common to encounter physical, psychological and medical conditions which impede the patient's ability to perform adequate home care and impact on the periodontal condition. Many older patients use several medications and they may be diagnosed with more than one chronic disease that can result in

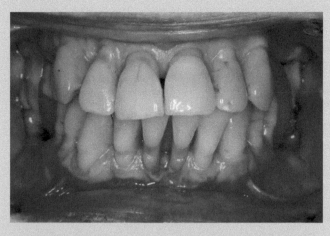

Figure 1.3.4 Patient after completion of non-surgical periodontal treatment.

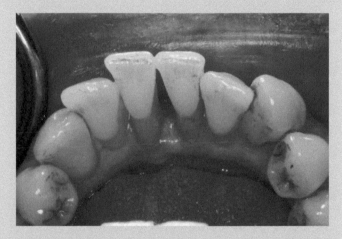

Figure 1.3.5 Lower incisors after removal of supragingival calculus deposits.

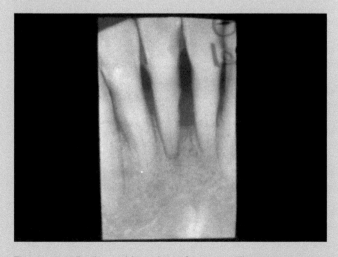

Figure 1.3.6 Radiographic review after 1 year illustrating no progression of horizontal bone loss association with lower incisors.

modifications to routine periodontal care. Moreover, chronic inflammatory diseases are common in older people, and the use of anti-inflammatory medications may have modulating effects on periodontal status, including evidence of plaque-induced gingival inflammation and periodontal pockets.

- The goal for treatment should be to preserve a functional, comfortable and aesthetically acceptable dentition. The basic treatment plan, encompassing non-surgical periodontal therapy supported by self-performed oral hygiene, is no different to that for a younger patient. Studies have shown that age is not a significant factor in determining outcome following treatment.[9]
- Similarly, age is not a contraindication to periodontal surgery, healing in older patients being no

different compared to younger individuals. The factors influencing the decision to undertake surgical intervention, including levels of plaque control and smoking, are the same in all age groups. Maintenance therapy is a key component of the comprehensive periodontal treatment plan, and its effectiveness has previously been demonstrated in patients treated for advanced periodontal disease.[9]

- Evidence for maintenance therapy specific to older individuals is limited, but one study found that in individuals between the ages of 60 and 96, those with regular dental visits retained more teeth; however, the frequency of dental visits had no impact on plaque deposits, gingival inflammation or alveolar bone levels.[8]

Self-Study Questions

1. Which probe is used to carry out a basic periodontal examination (BPE)?
   a. Williams probe
   b. World Health Organisation (WHO) BPE probe
   c. Sharp probe
   d. Furcation probe

2. Which of the following describes the clinical appearance of a BPE code 2?
   a. Furcation involvement
   b. Pocket depths <3.5 mm, supra- or subgingival calculus present
   c. Probing depth >5.5 mm
   d. Probing depth 3.5–5.5 mm

3. How is progression of attachment loss in older adults mainly seen clinically?
   a. Deepening periodontal pockets
   b. Gingival swelling
   c. Bleeding
   d. Gingival recession

4. Which of the following systemic conditions can have a negative impact on mechanical plaque control in older patients?
   a. Parkinson's disease
   b. Hypertension
   c. High cholesterol
   d. Angina

Answers are located at the end of the case

Self-Study Answers

1. b. World Health Organisation (WHO) BPE probe[10]

2. b. Pocket depths <3.5 mm, supra- or subgingival calculus present[10]

3. d. Gingival recession[5]

4. a. Parkinson's disease[5]

References

1 Locker D, Slade GD, Murray H (1998). Epidemiology of periodontal disease among older adults: a review. *Periodontology 2000* 16: 16–33.

2 Kiyak HA, Persson RE, Persson GR (1998). Influences on the perceptions of and responses to periodontal disease among older adults. *Periodontology 2000* 16: 34–43.

3 McArthur WP (1998). Effect of aging on immunocompetent and inflammatory cells. *Periodontology 2000* 16: 53–79.

4 Feres M, Teles F, Teles R, et al. (2016). The subgingival periodontal microbiota of the aging mouth. *Periodontology 2000* 72: 30–53.

5 Irwin CR (2011). Periodontal disease in the older patient. *Dental Update* 38: 94–100.

6 Allen PF, McKenna G, Creugers N (2011). Prosthodontic care for elderly patients. *Dental Update* 38: 460–470.

7 Hirschfeld L, Wasserman B. (1978) A long-term survey of tooth loss in 600 treated periodontal patients. *Journal of Periodontology* 49: 225–237.

8 Renvert S, Persson GR. (2016) Treatment of periodontal disease in older adults. *Periodontology 2000* 72: 108–119.

9 Lindhe J, Socransky S, Nyman S, et al. (1985). Effect of age on healing following periodontal therapy. *Journal of Clinical Periodontology* 12: 774–787.

10 British Society of Periodontology (2019). *Basic Periodontal Examination*. British Society of Periodontology, Liverpool.

Case 4

Splinting and Maintenance of Periodontally Involved Lower Incisors

With Contribution from Lewis Winning and Christopher Irwin

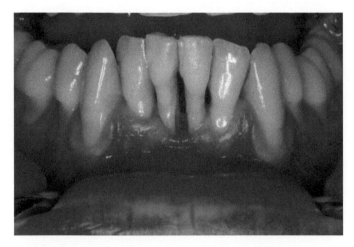

Figure 1.4.1 Lower incisor teeth at initial presentation.

A. Case Story

A 63-year-old male presented with loose lower incisors (Figure 1.4.1). He had been aware of increased mobility over the last three years, and was now conscious of looseness when eating. The patient's relevant medical history was clear and he was a non-smoker. He had previously had some non-surgical periodontal treatment of the lower incisor region and regularly attended his dental hygienist. A number of treatment options were discussed with the patient, including extraction of the mobile lower anterior teeth and prosthodontic replacement. The patient was very keen to retain his lower teeth for as long as possible even though they had a guarded long-term prognosis. Non-surgical periodontal treatment was carried out followed by splinting of the teeth.

LEARNING GOALS AND OBJECTIVES
- Understand that the aim of periodontal splinting is to improve masticatory function and comfort of teeth
- Identify when mobility in periodontally involved teeth has reached a level where functional

interference is apparent and then splinting of the teeth is indicated
- Recognise that splinting must be accompanied by adequate oral hygiene and maintenance, as mechanical cleaning of the teeth is compromised by the presence of the periodontal splint

B. Medical History
- Osteoarthritis
- Atrial fibrillation
- High blood pressure controlled by medication
- Irregular heart beat
- High cholesterol controlled by medication and diet
- Former smoker, quit 20 years ago

C. Dental History
- Regular dental attender
- No previous experience of removable prosthesis
- Previous treatment for periodontal disease with dental hygienist

D. Medications
- Warfarin (anticoagulant) 2 mg daily
- Aspirin (non-steroidal anti-inflammatory) 50 mg daily
- Propranolol hydrochloride (beta blocker) 80 mg twice per day
- Simvastatin (CoA reductase inhibitor) 40 mg once daily

E. Social History
- Retired, previous mechanic
- Previous smoker, quit approximately 20 years ago
- Alcohol: approximately 20 units per week

F. Extraoral Examination
- No significant findings

- Alcohol: approximately 10 units per week
- Lives with wife and has two adult children

F. Extraoral Examination

- Temporomandibular joint (TMJ): nothing abnormal detected, mouth opening normal
- Muscles of mastication: nothing abnormal detected
- Lymph nodes: nothing abnormal detected

G. Soft Tissue Examination

- No significant findings
- Extremely resorbed mandibular alveolar ridge, with limited keratinised oral mucosa
- No evidence of oral dryness detected intraorally

H. Clinical Findings/Problem List

- Patient is edentate in upper and lower arches
- In the upper jaw the posterior ridge was well formed, but the anterior alveolar bone had been replaced with mobile fibrous tissue. For this reason, the level of difficulty according to the American College of Prosthodontics Prosthodontic Diagnostic Index was classification 3[1]

- The old set of dentures the patient was wearing were poorly adapted and there were signs of ulceration associated with areas of overextension of the lower denture periphery
- The occlusal surfaces of the dentures were extremely worn, and the freeway space was measured at 12 mm
- The denture teeth were set in the neutral zone, and the polished surfaces of the dentures were classed as favourable
- The most recently provided set of dentures were extremely unretentive, particularly the upper denture. There was an premature contact in the centric relation position which produced a definite slide from the retruded contact position to the intercuspal position, and had a destabilising effect on the retention of the dentures

I. Diagnoses

- Patient is edentate in the upper and lower arches
- Unretentive and unstable dentures; excessive freeway space; complex presentation due to severe resorption and presence of mobile fibrous tissue in the maxilla

CLINICAL DECISION MAKING – DETERMINING FACTORS

- The patient is relatively young, and had until recently been successfully rehabilitated using complete replacement dentures. He is well disposed to complete replacement denture therapy, and is not seeking complex treatment involving dental implants. The prognosis for treatment is good, as he has managed to wear very worn and ill-fitting dentures for some time. However, care must be taken to avoid drastic changes when making him a new set of dentures. He has become accustomed to a large freeway space and the shape of the current polished surfaces. This was clearly not taken into account when making his most recent set of dentures, and the polished surfaces bore little resemblance to his older set. The major reduction in freeway space has also contributed to his rejection of the most recent set.
  - The condition of his denture-bearing area is challenging. Great care has to be taken when recording the master impressions in cases where there is mobile tissue/a flabby ridge. If this tissue is excessively compressed during impression making, then the

denture made from this impression will displace the underlying mobile tissue and render the denture unstable and unretentive. In this case, a selective pressure impression technique was used.[2] This involved:
  - Making a customised impression tray with a window overlying the anterior mobile tissue, but closely fitted to the denture-bearing area elsewhere (Figure 2.6.2).
  - Recording the master impression with zinc oxide and eugenol impression paste (Impression Paste, SS White, UK), following border moulding with green stick tracing compound.
  - Removing the paste from the window area, reseating the impression and applying impression plaster (Snow White™, Kerr Dental, USA) over the exposed mobile tissue (Figure 2.6.3).
  - Careful wrapping of the impression to protect the brittle plaster; disinfection prior to sending to the laboratory for casting.
- The significantly resorbed mandible makes it difficult to stabilise the record rim when recording

the jaw relationship. This, coupled with the fact that the patient has a habitual forward posture due to excessive freeway space, increases the difficulty in recording the jaw relationship in centric relation. In these circumstances, use of heat-cured acrylic bases for record rims should be considered with a view to increasing the stability of the rims (Figure 2.6.4). This made it easier to record an accurate jaw relationship record in this case.

- For this patient a decision needed to be made about how much freeway space change should be made, and how quickly it should be done. When considering how much it should be reduced by, consideration must be given to the impact a large reduction may have on denture stability and appearance. In this case, given the history of

intolerance of a very large change in freeway space, it was decided to reduce the freeway space gradually on the existing set of old dentures. Occlusal pivots were created by incremental addition of tooth-coloured self-cured acrylic resin (SNAP™, Parkell Inc., USA) over two clinical visits two weeks apart (Figure 2.6.5). This allowed the patient to adapt slowly to a gradual increase in occlusal vertical dimension (reduced freeway space), and made it easier to record the jaw relationship in centric relation. The patient tolerated this change well, with minimal adjustment. He also reported satisfaction with the impact on his appearance. Following this procedure, a decision was made to provide 6 mm of freeway space in his new dentures, a reduction of 6 mm from his existing freeway space. The impact on his appearance can be seen by comparing old and new dentures in situ (Figures 2.6.6 and 2.6.7).

- A combination of significant resorption and replacement of alveolar ridge with fibrous tissue creates

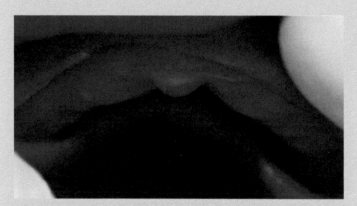

Figure 2.6.2 Open tray over 'flabby' anterior maxillary ridge.

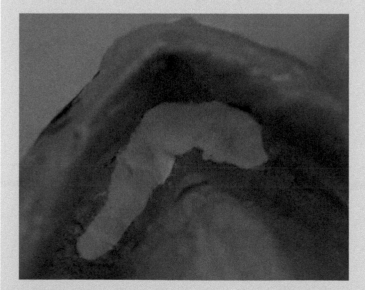

Figure 2.6.3 Master impression recorded using selective pressure impression technique.

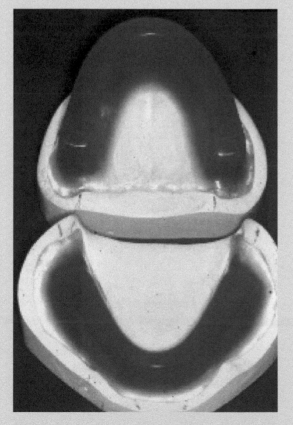

Figure 2.6.4 Record blocks with wax rims and permanent bases.

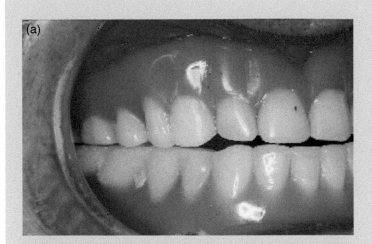

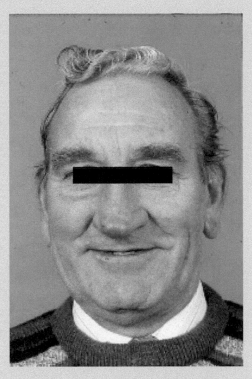

Figure 2.6.6 Pre-treatment view of patient with historical dentures in situ. Note the lack of visibility of maxillary anterior teeth when smiling.

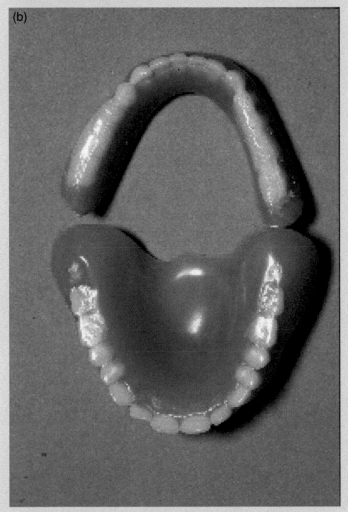

Figure 2.6.5 (a) and (b) Incremental build-up of occlusal surfaces of complete dentures using occlusal pivots; (a) buccal view; (b) occlusal view.

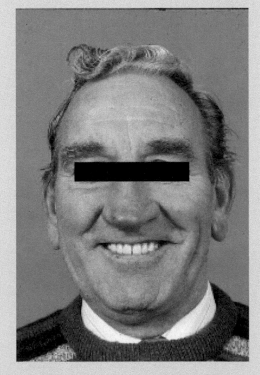

Figure 2.6.7 Post-treatment view with new dentures in situ.

challenges for both retention and stability. Consideration must be given to the occlusal scheme for dentures in these circumstances. Use of cuspless teeth or teeth with zero-degree cusp angles has its advantages in achieving balanced articulation, but impacts negatively on appearance and chewing function. It is essential to achieve balanced articulation in dynamic lateral and protrusive movements, and this is aided by use of a semi-adjustable articulator when mounting teeth.

This is not essential, but can reduce chairside adjustment time.

- Polished surface shape is highly influential in physiological retention of complete dentures. By this means, some patients overcome highly unfavourable anatomical presentations and manage to control their dentures in function. The 'copy denture' technique is a method for duplicating the existing polished surfaces and replicating them in the new dentures.

Self-Help Questions

1. Which of the following impression materials would be appropriate for taking a mucocompressive primary impression for complete dentures?
   a. Impression compound
   b. Plaster
   c. Light-bodied silicone
   d. Alginate

2. Which of the following is an anatomical landmark used to help determine the orientation of the occlusal plane during complete denture construction?
   a. Mental foramen
   b. Midline of face
   c. Ala-tragus line
   d. Interpupillary line

3. Which sort of occlusal relationship should be prescribed when constructing complete dentures?
   a. Canine guidance
   b. Group function
   c. Balanced articulation
   d. Posterior disclusion

Answers are located at the end of the case

Self-Help Answers

1. a. Impression compound

2. c. Ala-tragus line

3. c. Balanced articulation

References

1 McGarry TJ, Nimmo A, Skibo JF, et al. (1999). Classification system for complete edentulism. The American College of Prosthodontics. *Journal of Prosthodontics* 8: 27–39.

2 Lynch CD, Allen PF (2006). Management of the flabby ridge: using contemporary materials to solve an old problem. *British Dental Journal* 200: 258–261.

Case 7

Fabrication of New Complete Replacement Dentures Using a Copy Technique

With Contribution from Gerry McKenna, Robert Thompson and Claudio Leles

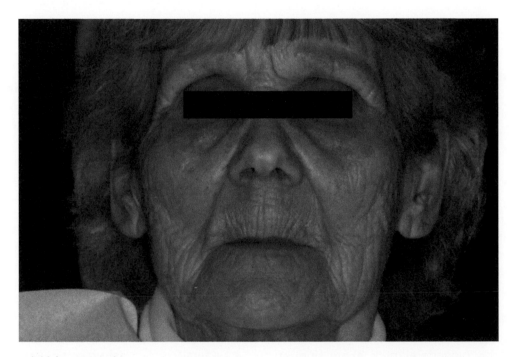

Figure 2.7.1 Patient at initial presentation.

A. Case Story

A 79-year-old female was referred to a dental school for provision of new dentures. The patient had no remaining natural teeth and had been wearing dentures for over 40 years. She was very pleased with the aesthetics of her existing dentures, but felt that the retention was becoming less on the upper prosthesis. She did not report any significant functional issues, but did want to have more teeth on show (Figure 2.7.1). The patient had been provided with a new set of conventional dentures approximately two years beforehand, but had been unable to accommodate to them and felt that they were 'very different' to her current set. The dentures that she was wearing at presentation were around 5 years old.

LEARNING GOALS AND OBJECTIVES
- Appreciate that complete replacement dentures can be fabricated using a conventional or copy technique; understand when these techniques are indicated
- Understand that careful case selection for the copy technique is vitally important; the copy technique can be utilised where the existing prostheses are well constructed and require a relatively small amount of modification
- Appreciate that where significant denture faults exist such as large occlusal errors or errors in tooth position, then the conventional technique is more appropriate

- Recognise that as the copy technique combines both major impressions and jaw registration, it can be completed in less clinical time; it also provides significant psychological advantages to the patient, as accommodation and adaptation to the new dentures may be more easily achieved[1, 2]

B. Medical History

- Osteoarthritis
- Atrial fibrillation
- High cholesterol
- Anxiety controlled by medication

C. Dental History

- Edentulous for 43 years
- The patient had all her teeth removed and immediate dentures fitted 43 years ago
- The patient has worn complete dentures successfully for many years
- Her current set of dentures are five years old and the patient is very pleased with the aesthetics, although she would like to 'show more of her teeth'
- She finds that the lower denture moves in function and food is becoming trapped underneath
- The patient does not wish to consider more complex options such as dental implants

D. Medications

- Warfarin (anticoagulant) 3 mg daily (target INR 2.5, monitored monthly by general medical practitioner)
- Aspirin (non-steroidal anti-inflammatory) 150 mg daily
- Ibuprofen gel (non-steroidal anti-inflammatory) as required
- Diazepam (benzodiazepine) 10 mg once daily

E. Social History

- Widowed, lives with daughter and her family
- Her daughter accompanies her to all appointments
- Previously worked as a schoolteacher
- Non-smoker
- Alcohol: less than 5 units per week

F. Extraoral Examination

- Temporomandibular joint (TMJ): asymptomatic click on right side, no evidence of limited opening
- Muscles of mastication: nothing abnormal detected
- Lymph nodes: nothing abnormal detected

G. Soft Tissue Examination

- No significant findings

H. Clinical Findings/Problem List

- Edentate upper and lower arch
- Resorbed maxillary and mandibular ridges, no evidence of mobile/flabby tissue in either arch
- The existing dentures were well adapted but slightly underextended; the upper denture did not extend to the full height of the functional sulcus
- The denture teeth were worn but not excessively
- The incisal level provided little teeth on show; the patient indicated that she wanted to show more of her upper teeth
- The dentures appeared to provide appropriate lip support

I. Diagnosis

- Patient is edentate in the upper and lower arches
- Generally well-constructed but worn complete dentures; patient is happy with the aesthetics, including tooth position, mould and shade, but would like to have a more retentive set constructed with more upper teeth on show

CLINICAL DECISION MAKING – DETERMINING FACTORS

- The patient has been wearing complete replacement dentures for over 40 years and has successfully adapted to removable prostheses. She does not wish to consider more complex options, including implant-retained overdentures or fixed implant bridges. She wishes to have new removable dentures constructed.

- Complete denture construction can be undertaken using two clinical approaches: conventional technique and the copy technique.
- The patient's existing dentures have been well constructed and she is very happy with most aspects of them. The dentures are well extended and although the teeth are worn, tooth position, occlusion and aesthetics are all correct.

- Although the patient did not bring her most recently constructed set of dentures to any appointments, her description would indicate that these were very different in a number of ways to her existing dentures. As a result, she had been unable to accommodate to them and had returned them to the dentist who constructed them.
- In order to minimise the changes in the new dentures, it was decided to utilise the copy denture technique to construct them.
- The patient's existing dentures were copied using putty (Lab-Putty, Coltene, UK) placed in large impression trays (Figure 2.7.2). Vaseline was used to ensure that the putty could be separated and the denture removed. This was repeated for the upper and lower prostheses.

- Upper and lower wax copies of the dentures were fabricated and returned to the clinic. Wash impressions were taken in the wax copies using light-bodied silicone (Take 1™ Advanced™, Kerr, USA) and a jaw registration was performed.
- A denture try-in was completed and when the clinician and patient were both happy, the dentures were sent to the lab for completion (Figure 2.7.3).
- The final dentures were completed and fitted (Figure 2.7.4).
- The copy technique used in this case offered significant psychological advantages to the patient and ensured that minimal accommodation was required once the new dentures were fitted.

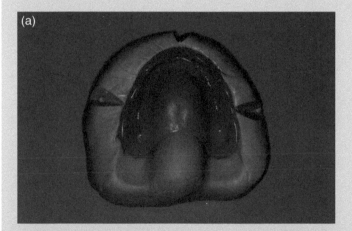

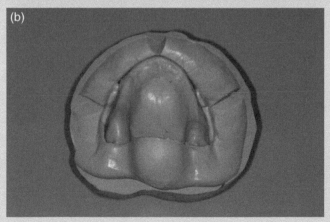

Figure 2.7.2 (a) and (b) Putty impression of existing upper denture (Lab-Putty, Coltene™, UK).

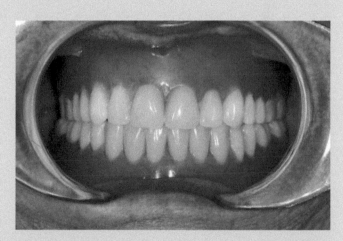

Figure 2.7.3 Denture try-in.

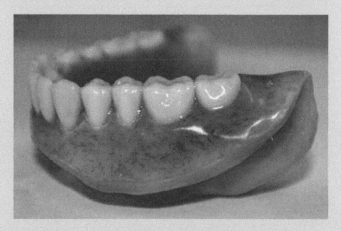

Figure 2.7.4 Completed full lower denture.

- The technique was completed more quickly than a conventional technique, as the stages of major impressions and jaw registration were combined.
- The copy technique was utilised very successfully in this case; however, careful case selection is vitally important. The copy technique was chosen for this patient as her existing dentures were well constructed and required a relatively small amount of modification. Where significant denture faults exist such as large occlusal errors or errors in tooth position, then the copy technique is not recommended. Clinicians should only copy dentures that are worth copying.
- Although not used in this case, modifications to existing dentures should be completed prior to undertaking the copy technique. For example, where dentures are underextended, greenstick compound can be added to the peripheries to improve the extensions and then the modified denture copied in putty.

Self-Study Questions

1. Which clinical stages can be combined during the construction of copy dentures?
    a. Primary and secondary impressions
    b. Try-in and fit
    c. Secondary impression and jaw registration
    d. Jaw registration and try-in

2. Compared to conventional denture construction, how long will fabrication of copy dentures take?
    a. The same amount of time
    b. Less time
    c. More time

3. Which materials can be used to make a copy impression of a patient's existing denture?
    a. Alginate
    b. Impression compound
    c. Silicone putty
    d. Impression plaster

Answers are located at the end of the case

Self-Study Answers

1. c. Secondary impression and jaw registration

2. b. Less time

3. a. Alginate and c. Silicone putty

References

1 Mohamed TJ, Faraj SA (2001). Duplication of complete dentures using a sectional mould technique. *Journal of Prosthetic Dentistry* 85: 12–14.

2 Kippax A, Watson CJ, Basker RM, Pentland JE (1998). How well are complete dentures copied? *British Dental Journal* 185: 129–133.

Case 8

Provision of Upper and Lower Implant-Retained Overdentures for an Older Patient

With Contribution from Harald Gjengedal, Finbarr Allen, Martin Schimmel and Murali Srinivasan

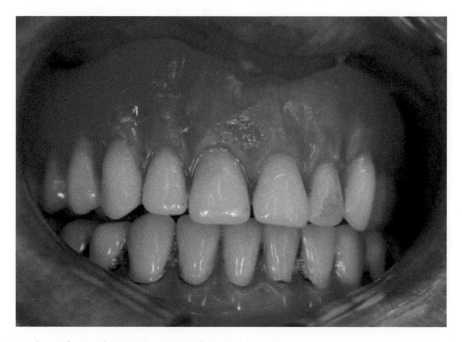

Figure 2.8.1 Pre-treatment view of complete replacement dentures.

A. Case Story

A frail 85-year-old female presented for treatment. She had been edentulous for over 50 years and was wearing upper and lower removable complete prostheses. Her current maxillary denture was one year old, but she has never been satisfied with the function of the denture. She reported that the lack of retention and stability were making chewing and speaking very difficult. She also reported that she was experiencing problems in finding a 'comfortable biting position' (Figure 2.8.1). She was, however, satisfied with the aesthetics of the maxillary denture. Because of these problems the patient felt that she had lost weight and had become depressed. Her husband accompanied her to the clinic and confirmed that the patient had withdrawn from her usual social engagements. The patient and her husband were informed by the referring dentist that the current dentures could not

be improved. After consideration of a number of treatment options, the patient was successfully rehabilitated using upper and lower implant-retained overdentures.

LEARNING GOALS AND OBJECTIVES
- Appreciate that dental implants can be used to support complete removable dentures in both the mandible and maxilla
- Recognise that it is widely accepted that restoration of the edentulous mandible with a conventional denture is no longer the most appropriate first-choice prosthodontic treatment; there is now overwhelming evidence that a two-implant overdenture should become the first-choice treatment for the edentulous mandible[1]

- Understand that fundamental prosthodontic principles must still be followed when designing and constructing an implanted-supported overdenture
- Remember that age is not a barrier to implant treatment, as implant prostheses in older adults are a predictable treatment option with very high survival rates reported[2, 3]

B. Medical History

- Patient is visibly frail
- Asthma
- Rheumatoid arthritis
- Failing eyesight
- Patient is living independently with minimal assistance from her husband

C. Dental History

- The patient is an experienced denture wearer and has coped well with her conventional removable dentures up to the last few years
- She had a complete replacement upper denture constructed approximately one year ago, but this has not been successful; the patient finds the upper denture unretentive and uncomfortable to wear; she applies a large amount of denture adhesive to the upper denture
- The present mandibular denture is over 10 years old

D. Medications

- Salbutamol (bronchodilator) 100 mcg up to four times daily
- Diclofenac (non-steroidal anti-inflammatory) 75 mg twice daily
- Diazepam (benzodiazepine) 10 mg once daily
- Aspirin (non-steroidal anti-inflammatory) 150 mg daily
- Calcium carbonate (dietary supplement) 500 mg twice daily
- Allergy to penicillin

E. Social History

- Patient is retired, previously worked as a teacher
- Lives with her husband
- Smokes approximately 10 cigarettes per day
- Does not drink alcohol

F. Extraoral Examination

- Temporomandibular joint (TMJ): nothing abnormal detected, mouth opening slightly limited
- Muscles of mastication: nothing abnormal detected
- Lymph nodes: nothing abnormal detected

G. Soft Tissue Examination

- No significant findings

H. Clinical Findings/Problem List

- The mandibular alveolar ridge was very resorbed, small and thin
- The maxillary alveolar ridge was even more resorbed, the anterior part of the ridge was extremely resorbed but not particularly mobile; posteriorly the tuberosities were particularly prominent, hanging down over 1 cm below the level of the anterior alveolar ridge (Figure 2.8.2a and b)
- The maxillary denture was extremely unstable and unretentive; the denture was overextended in the periphery and there was no stable interocclusal relationship; the occlusal contacts were not evenly distributed and there was a premature contact on the left side; thus it was difficult for the patient to find a stable occlusal contact
- The mandibular denture was worn and discoloured; the entire maxillary denture was suboptimally polished and felt rough

I. Diagnosis

- The patient is completely edentulous
- Severe alveolar ridge resorption in both jaws
- Prominent maxillary tuborosities
- Unretentive and unstable existing complete dentures

CLINICAL DECISION MAKING – DETERMINING FACTORS

- The patient was an experienced denture wearer. However, the problematic new maxillary denture had a significant negative impact on her quality of life. She was in desperate need of help; her husband felt she just 'vanished' in front of him. Being told by her former dentist that the dentures could not be improved worsened her mental and physical condition. Therefore it was of the utmost importance to increase the retention and stability of her dentures.
- The prominent tuberosities had a negative influence on the retention and stability of the maxillary denture.

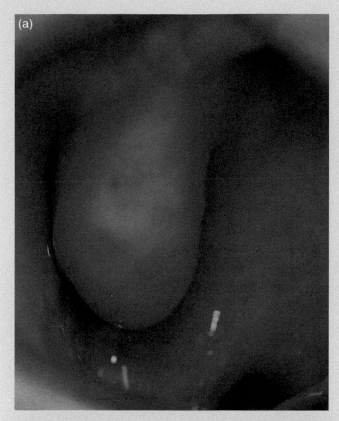

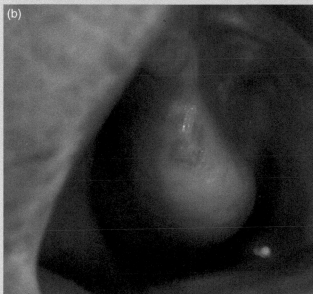

Figure 2.8.2 (a) Right tuberosity region: note the extensive bulk of soft tissue, which was mobile and extended vertically; (b) left tuberosity region: similar bulk of mobile soft tissue to the right side.

They were also having a negative impact on the tooth position and vertical height of the denture. Surgical excision of the fibrous tissue in this region was needed to level the alveolar ridge and create more interalveolar ridge space.

- Both dentures were unstable and unretentive. As the alveolar ridges were significantly resorbed, it was decided that the best way to increase stability and retention was using implant-retained prostheses. Radiographic examination indicated sufficient alveolar bone height in the mandible for two implants in the canine position (Figure 2.8.3). In the maxilla, however, only 4–7 mm of bone height was available, making implant placement more challenging.
- The following treatment plan was developed with the patient:
  - Excision of fibrous tissues in the posterior maxilla.
  - Relining of the maxillary denture with soft material in the early healing phase.
  - Regular relining and reshaping of both dentures.
  - Placement of implants in the mandible.
  - Placement of implants in the maxilla.
  - Construction of new implant overdentures and attachment using locator abutments.
- The objective of this treatment plan was to make the dentures functional as soon as possible.
- The fibrous tissue was excised and two weeks later the maxillary denture was relined with soft relining material (GC Reline™ Soft, GC Corporation, Japan). After two weeks the dentures were reshaped and an impression was made with polyether (Impregum™, 3M, USA) and the dentures relined chairside with a hard material (GC Reline™, GC Corporation, Japan).

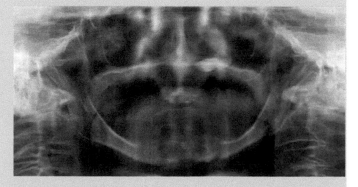

Figure 2.8.3 Pre-treatment orthopantomograph (OPG). Note the lack of bone in the maxilla.

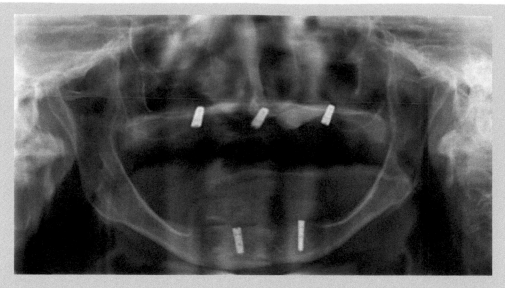

Figure 2.8.4 Post-surgical orthopantomograph (OPG) showing the implants placed. The middle implant in the maxilla failed to osseointegrate and was removed at second-stage surgery.

- Two bone-level implants (3.3 × 10 mm; Straumann Roxolid, Switzerland) were placed in the mandible under local anaesthetic.
- 10 days later three bone-level implants (3.3 × 8 mm; Straumann Roxolid, Switzerland) were placed in the maxilla under local anaesthetic (Figure 2.8.4). The implants had suboptimal primary stability and therefore a delayed loading protocol was decided upon. Both dentures were adjusted postoperatively.
- Two months after implant installation, a new mandibular denture was made. The patient was satisfied with the aesthetic of the maxillary denture and did not want a new denture constructed for financial reasons.
- Three months after implant placement in the mandible, the second-stage surgery was carried out under local anaesthetic. Five days later the locator abutments were attached and the retentive elements were directly mounted in the new denture with self-curing acrylic (Quick Up, Voco, USA) (Figure 2.8.5).
- Eight months after implant installation in the maxilla, the second-stage surgery was completed under local anaesthetic. The reason for this

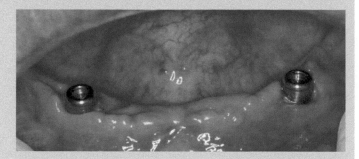

Figure 2.8.5 Locator™ (Zest Dental Systems, USA) abutments in situ, favourable angulation.

prolonged healing period was the suboptimal primary stability of the implants. Unfortunately, the implant in midline had not osseointegrated and was removed. Two weeks after the operation the Locator™ (Zest Dental Systems, USA) abutments were attached and the retentive elements mounted in the denture using self-curing acrylic (Quick Up, Voco, USA) (Figures 2.8.6 and 2.8.7a and b).
- The increased retention and stability of the dentures had a dramatic impact on the patient and her everyday life, including her social interactions (Figure 2.8.8a and b).

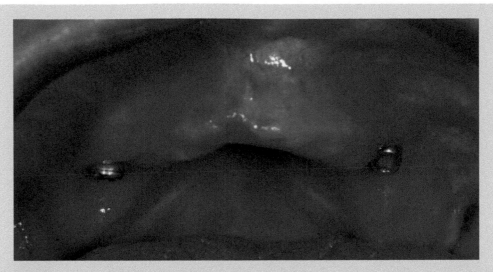

Figure 2.8.6 Locator™ (Zest Dental Systems, USA) abutments in situ. Note the mesial angulation of the left abutment. This required Locator cap is designed to manage up to 20° angulation of abutment.

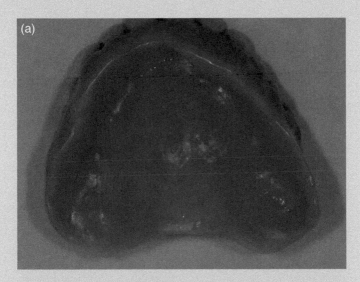

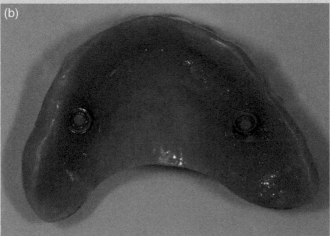

Figure 2.8.7 (a) Fitting surface of new complete replacement denture prior to the insertion of Locator caps; (b) fitting surface of new complete replacement denture following chairside processing of Locator caps into the base.

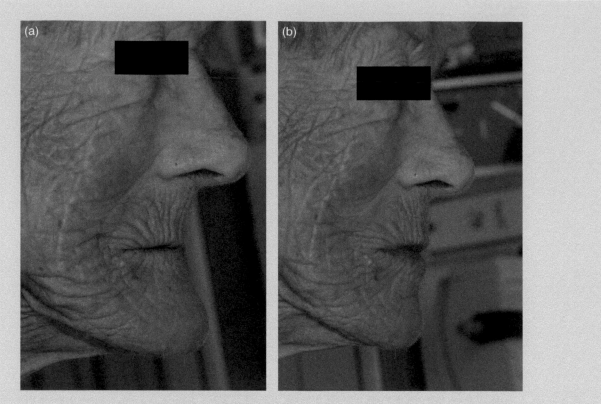

Figure 2.8.8 Lateral views (a) pre treatment; (b) post treatment.

Self-Study Questions

1. In frail edentate patients, what is the best form of implant-retained or supported prosthesis?
   a. One that is easy to remove
   b. One that is fixed in place
   c. One that is easy to remove and clean
   d. One that has the most pleasing appearance

2. What do overdentures retained on two implants require?
   a. A suitable band of keratinised tissue around each implant
   b. Implants to be placed 30 mm apart
   c. Magnets to retain the denture
   d. A bar to be placed between the implants

3. What are the options for retentive components to attach an overdenture to dental implants?
   a. Studs/balls
   b. Magnets
   c. Bar
   d. Milled crowns

Answers are located at the end of the case

Self-Study Answers

1. c. One that is easy to remove and clean

2. a. A suitable band of keratinised tissue around each implant

3. a. Studs/balls, b. Magnets and c. Bar.

References

1 Feine JS (2002). The McGill consensus statement on over-dentures. *Mandibular two-implant overdentures as first choice standard of care for edentulous patients. International Journal of Maxillofacial Implants* 17: 601–602.
2 Schimmel M, Srinivasan M, McKenna G, Müller F (2018). Effect of advanced age and/or systemic medical conditions on dental implant survival: a systematic review and meta-analysis. *Clinical Oral Implants Research* 16: 311–330.
3 Heitz-Mayfield LJ, Aaboe M, Araujo M, et al. (2018). Group 4 ITI consensus report: risks and biologic complications associated with implant dentistry. *Clinical Oral Implants Research* 16: 351–358.

Case 9

Use of a Removable Partial Denture to Replace Missing Teeth

With Contribution from Finbarr Allen

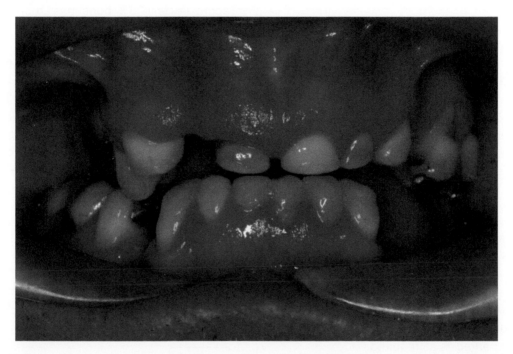

Figure 2.9.1 Note the first point of contact (RCP) between 14 and 45. This is a useful reference point for planning the final intercuspal position (ICP). Prior to treatment, the patient had a horizontal anterior slide into ICP.

A. Case Story

A 67-year-old male with a history of worn anterior teeth, a loose upper removable partial denture and repeated fracture of anterior restorations presented for treatment (Figure 2.9.1). He was dissatisfied with the appearance of his upper anterior teeth and reported problems with chewing efficiency. He had been partially dentate in both jaws for over 20 years, and had noticed his upper teeth getting 'shorter' in recent years. Repeated attempts to increase the size of the teeth with adhesive restorations had failed. He was wearing a mucosa-borne acrylic removable partial denture at the time of presentation, but reported that it was loose and he had resorted to use of denture adhesive to help retain it.

LEARNING GOALS AND OBJECTIVES
- Understand that management of cases without a stable intercuspal position (ICP) requires significant planning and assessment prior to undertaking treatment
- Appreciate that where a stable ICP is not present, then use of retruded contact position (RCP) is indicated. This represents a reproducible, anatomical position where the first tooth contact is detected when the mandible is moving in the terminal hinge axis. Use of RCP may also create interocclusal space for restorations, as the RCP–ICP slide is eliminated

- Recognise that it can be challenging to record RCP in some patients and the use of a hard acrylic splint for a period time may be indicated to facilitate this

B. Medical History

- Patient reported no immediate health concerns, but attended his general medical practitioner for regular check-ups
- High blood pressure
- High cholesterol
- Patient had a history of gastric reflux, which he controlled using over-the-counter antacids

C. Dental History

- Partially dentate for approximately 20 years, with most recent dental extraction approximately 5 years ago
- Has had two sets of upper acrylic partial dentures constructed, but had never worn a lower denture
- Is an irregular dental attender, but has attended frequently in recent times to repair fractured anterior composite resin restorations over the past two years

D. Medications

- Aspirin (non-steroidal anti-inflammatory) 150 mg daily
- Propranolol hydrochloride (beta blocker) 80 mg twice daily
- Simvastatin (CoA reductase inhibitor) 40 mg once daily
- Atenolol (beta blocker) 50 mg twice daily
- Over-the-counter antacids as required

E. Social History

- Married with grown-up children
- Retired carpenter
- Non-smoker
- Alcohol: approximately 10 units per week (beer)

F. Extraoral Examination

- Temporomandibular joint (TMJ): nothing abnormal detected, mouth opening normal
- Muscles of mastication: nothing abnormal detected, but some tenderness associated with masseter on right side
- Lymph nodes: nothing abnormal detected

G. Soft Tissue Examination

- Linea alba on right and left buccal mucosa
- Bilateral tongue scalloping

H. Clinical Findings/Problem List

- The patient has a heavily restored posterior dentition, but no active caries
- His standard of oral hygiene is fair, but there has been approximately 30% bone loss around his anterior and posterior teeth; gingival recession is evident around his maxillary molar teeth
- His anterior teeth are short, consistent with a pattern of attritional toothwear (Figure 2.9.1)
- His lower anterior incisal edges have been restored with directly placed composite resin restoration, which is jagged and uneven; the patient reports that this causes trauma to his tongue on occasion
- He has had endodontic treatment of #11 and 22; he has no reproducible ICP; there is a freeway space of 7 mm
- His acrylic removable partial denture is loose and unstable, with evidence of mucosal trauma in the #12 area
- Tooth charting:

			4	3	2	1	1		3			6	7	
	7	6	5		3	2	1	1	2	3				

- Basic periodontal examination:

–	2	2
2	2	–

I. Diagnoses

- Partially dentate in upper and lower arch
- Loose, unretentive upper partial denture
- Attritional toothwear affecting anterior teeth
- Unstable occlusion
- Chronic, moderate generalised periodontal disease

CLINICAL DECISION MAKING – DETERMINING FACTORS

- There is an unstable occlusion complicated by a large number of missing posterior units. This is causing trauma to his anterior teeth and loss of maxillary anterior restorations.
- There are no retentive features on the patient's existing mucosa-borne removable partial denture. This is exacerbated by the relatively short anterior abutment teeth. His denture is poorly supported

anteriorly and displaces easily under occlusal load. This is traumatising the periodontal tissues in the 11 and 13 regions.

- Upper and lower prostheses are required to stabilise the occlusion. The patient's RCP is between teeth #14 and 45 (Figure 2.9.1), and there is 4 mm of freeway space in this position. This allows sufficient room to provide an aesthetically acceptable restoration using this reference position. It is unlikely that there would be any issue with the patient being able to tolerate this change in occlusal face height, as it is within the 5 mm range of tolerance. However, it is sometimes difficult to accurately record the RCP when the patient has had an unstable occlusion for a prolonged period of time. In these circumstances, it is worth providing a stabilising occlusal splint (Figure 2.9.2). This is worn full time and adjusted periodically over a 4–6-week period until a reproducible, even occlusal contact on the splint is achieved and the patient is comfortable with the degree of opening from the previous ICP. It may

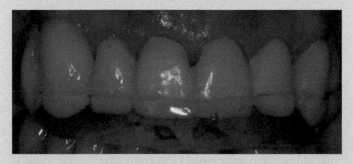

Figure 2.9.2 Bite-raising appliance (splint) in centric relation.

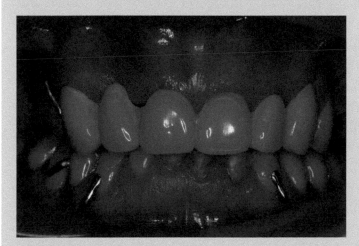

Figure 2.9.3 Anterior view of definitive overlay maxillary removable partial denture (RPD) and mandibular RPD.

also assist in determining the final appearance of anterior teeth, which will be longer that what the patient is accustomed to.

- The appearance of the patient's anterior teeth is not satisfactory. The situation is unfavourable for full-veneer crown restorations, as the teeth are short and offer poor retentive form. Directly placed composite resin restorations could be used when sufficient space has been created for them. However, teeth #11 and 22 will required non-vital bleaching to improve the possibilities for shade matching. A further option is to use a removable overlay approach, and use the short anterior teeth to support an overlay denture (Figure 2.9.3).
- Upper and lower removable partial dentures are indicated in this case given the multiple missing units. There is an extensive unilateral unbounded saddle in the left side of the mandible, which is potentially unfavourable. The patient has not previously had a lower denture, which is a further negative prognostic indicator. However, should the patient exhibit poor tolerance of a mandibular removable prosthesis, then the tooth position on the denture can be used to guide planning of an implant-retained prosthesis at a later date. A functionally orientated approach using the shortened dental arch concept could also be considered, but this is not a good option when the patient has an unstable occlusion and a dental arch shortened to the canine teeth on one or both sides.
- The patient has a history of chronic periodontal disease, and this must be stabilised using non-surgical management and customised oral hygiene advice prior to providing any rehabilitation. Cobalt-chromium alloy frameworks for removable partial dentures offer the possibility of reduced coverage of teeth, periodontal support tissues and oral mucosa when compared with acrylic resin-based denture. The design of frameworks for removable partial dentures must be undertaken to minimise the burden of plaque control. Components of the frameworks should be designed using hygienic principles.[1]
- Give the history of occlusal trauma, it is wise to protect the anterior acrylic resin teeth by extending the major connector onto the palatal aspect of the replacement teeth (Figure 2.9.4). When planning this, it is vital to determine the anterior tooth position in advance of making the framework. In this case, this was achieved by taking an impression of

stabilising splint in position and asking the dental technician to make an anterior tooth set-up based on this tooth position. The anterior teeth were set up in wax on the master model, which had been mounted against the mandibular cast in RCP. This was tried in the patient's mouth and necessary modifications made. Once an acceptable tooth position was determined, this was indexed using

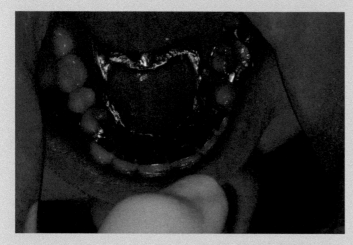

Figure 2.9.4 Occlusal view of maxillary overlay prosthesis. Note the metal backings protecting the anterior teeth.

laboratory putty (Figure 2.9.5). The indexed tooth position was then used as a guide when waxing the framework, thus ensuring that the inclination of the metal backings allowed sufficient space for the acrylic resin teeth.

- The framework should also be designed in such a way to allow addition of teeth to the framework at a subsequent date. For example, the periodontal support of tooth #11 was compromised, and its prognosis was guarded. The design of the overlay and framework allows easy adaptation of the denture in the event that #11 had to be extracted at a future date.
- The edges of the lower anterior teeth were jagged and uneven prior to treatment. On the mounted casts (described earlier), a diagnostic wax-up was undertaken to create an even inclination of the mandibular anterior teeth in even contact with the upper denture teeth trial denture. This was indexed using impression putty. The index was adapted to the teeth in the mouth (Figure 2.9.6) and used to aid direct placement of resin composite (CeramX Universal™, Dentsply, USA).

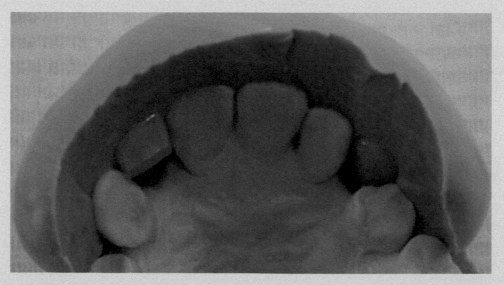

Figure 2.9.5 Index of desired anterior tooth position. This is used on the master cast when making the metal backings on the cobalt-chromium framework.

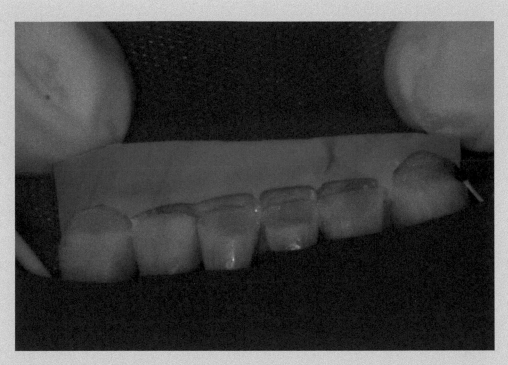

Figure 2.9.6 Putty index made on diagnostic wax-up cast, used to guide positioning and incremental build-up of composite resin restorations on mandibular anterior teeth.

Self-Study Questions

1. In patients with missing and worn teeth, what should the clinician do?
   a. Always conform to the existing intercuspal position
   b. Increase the occluding vertical dimension using removable dentures
   c. Increase the occluding vertical dimension using the natural teeth only
   d. Increase the occluding vertical dimension evenly on both denture and natural teeth

2. In toothwear cases, which of the following is most correct?
   a. Flowable composite resin is suitable for worn surfaces in attrition cases
   b. A minimum of 1 mm thickness of composite resin is required to restore worn surfaces
   c. A minimum of 2 mm thickness of composite resin is required to restore worn surfaces
   d. Indirect composite resin is the best material for this purpose

3. In older adults, which is pathogenic toothwear most likely to be caused by?
   a. Excessive tooth brushing
   b. Combination of erosion and attrition
   c. Gastric reflux
   d. Occlusal overload

Answers are located at the end of the case

Self-Study Answers

1. d. Increase the occluding vertical dimension evenly on both denture and natural teeth

2. c. A minimum of 2 mm thickness of composite resin is required to restore worn surfaces[2]

3. b. Combination of erosion and attrition[3]

References

1 Allen PF, McKenna G, Creugers N (2011). Prosthodontic care for elderly patients. *Dental Update* 38: 460–470.

2 Milosovic A, Burnside G (2016). The survival of composite restorations in the management of severe toothwear including attrition and erosion: a prospective 8-year study. *Journal of Dentistry* 44: 13–19.

3 Burke FM, McKenna G (2011). Toothwear and the older patient. *Dental Update* 38: 165–168.

Case 10

Integrating Fixed and Removable Prosthodontics

With Contribution from Conor McLister and Simon Killough

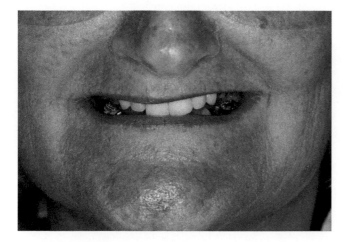

Figure 2.10.1 The patient's appearance at initial presentation.

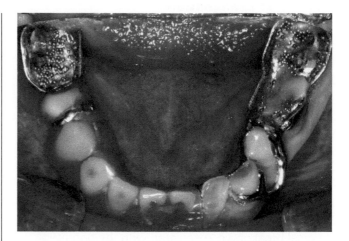

Figure 2.10.2 The patient's worn lower removable partial denture.

A. Case Story

A 66-year-old female presented with concerns regarding the appearance of worn teeth on her lower removable partial denture (RPD) (Figures 2.10.1 and 2.10.2). This prosthesis had been made approximately 15 years earlier, and the patient had noticed a significant deterioration in the last few years. In the maxilla, following recent extractions, she was wearing an acrylic RPD. This had an uneven anterior occlusal plane and was underextended palatally. She had a history of hypodontia and had been wearing a lower removable prosthesis for over 40 years. The patient wanted to have her upper and lower RPDs replaced with some more aesthetic prostheses.

LEARNING GOALS AND OBJECTIVES

- Understand that many treatment options are available to replace missing teeth, including fixed and removable prosthodontics
- Appreciate that when removable prosthodontics are planned, heavily restored abutment teeth can be utilised to provide retention for the partial denture through the use of extracoronal restorations
- Recognise that appropriate treatment planning is vitally important to ensure that extracoronal restorations are provided to facilitate the partial denture design

B. Medical History

- History of heart palpitations
- Well controlled diabetes mellitus

C. Dental History

- Patient reported tooth brushing twice daily with a fluoride toothpaste, but no interdental cleaning
- She removed her RPDs after meals for cleaning, but did not remove them at night
- The patient has been wearing RPDs successfully for over 40 years; she is not interested in exploring more complex treatment options and would like to have her RPDs replaced

CHAPTER 2

D. Medications
- Propranolol hydrochloride (beta blocker) 80 mg twice daily
- Simvastatin (CoA reductase inhibitor) 40 mg once daily
- Aspirin (non-steroidal anti-inflammatory) 75 mg once daily
- Multivitamins

E. Social History
- Married with grown-up children
- Provides childcare for grandchildren twice weekly
- Non-smoker
- Does not consume alcohol

F. Extraoral Examination
- Temporomandibular joint (TMJ): nothing abnormal detected
- Muscles of mastication: nothing abnormal detected
- Lymph nodes: nothing abnormal detected

G. Soft Tissue Examination
- No significant findings

H. Clinical Findings/Problem List
- Partially dentate in upper and lower arches (Figure 2.10.3)
- Generalised gingival recession
- Marginal breakdown associated with the porcelain bonded to metal crowns on both central incisors
- In the mandible there was significant residual ridge resorption; both lower first molars had large amalgam restorations with marginal breakdown (Figure 2.10.4); the lower left first molar was non-responsive to thermal vitality testing
- The lower left second molar had an existing amalgam restoration, but extensive secondary caries, and was non-responsive to thermal vitality testing

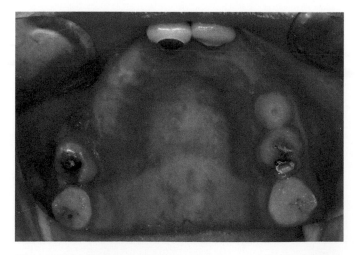

Figure 2.10.3 Palatal view of upper teeth.

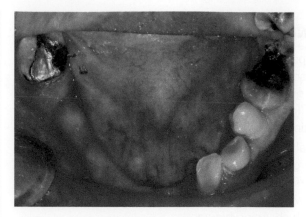

Figure 2.10.4 Residual lower dentition.

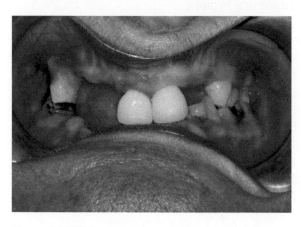

Figure 2.10.5 The patient's occlusion.

- There was incisal toothwear extending into dentine on the lower left lateral incisor and lower left canine; both of these teeth were Grade I mobile
- Occlusal analysis revealed an existing intercuspal position (ICP), with contacts posteriorly; there was a deep overbite and significantly reduced occlusal vertical dimension in relation to the vertical dimension at rest (Figure 2.10.5)
- Tooth charting:

	7	6				1	1			5	6	7	
		6						3	4	5	6	7	

- Basic periodontal examination:

2	2	2
–	2	2

I. Diagnoses
- Moderate chronic periodontitis
- Secondary caries
- Toothwear due to attrition
- Marginal breakdown of indirect restorations
- Partially edentate maxilla and mandible

CLINICAL DECISION MAKING – DETERMINING FACTORS

The patient was not experiencing any acute symptoms and so appropriate oral and denture hygiene advice was given. This included the use of interdental cleaning aids (Interdental brushes, TePe, UK) and removal of her existing prostheses at night time.

- Stabilisation treatment included a course of non-surgical periodontal treatment, including root surface debridement under local anaesthetic. The crowns in the upper central incisors were replaced with chairside bis-acrylic composite temporary crowns, and the margins were modified to allow improved oral hygiene.

- Failing restorations and secondary caries were removed in the lower first molar teeth. Caries extended into the pulp of the lower left first molar. As a terminal end abutment, this tooth was considered strategically important so endodontic treatment was completed (Figure 2.10.6). The lower left molar had extensive caries distally and was deemed unrestorable.

- As the patient had previous satisfactory denture experience, it was decided to consider replacement removable prostheses, using fixed restorations on abutment teeth to enhance retention, support and stability.

- Study models mounted on a semi-adjustable articular were analysed and options for restoring the vertical dimension of occlusion were discussed. These included maintaining the existing ICP and providing removable partial onlay dentures. However, the patient's existing onlay denture had worn significantly, and it was felt that stable tooth–tooth contacts could be achieved at an increased occlusal vertical dimension, using a combination of direct and indirect fixed restorations.

- A diagnostic mock-up of remaining teeth was fabricated at the planned new occlusal vertical dimension, and the models were surveyed to plan partial denture design.[1] From this, direct and indirect restorations on abutment teeth were planned to facilitate the denture design.

- Both of the mandibular terminal abutment teeth were restored with composite resin cores. Following core placement, it was decided to restore the endodontically treated lower left first molar and the lower right first molar with cast gold full-coverage crowns. Cast gold restorations are considered the most durable for posterior teeth, with type III or IV gold alloys used in high stress-bearing areas.[2]

- In this case, the path of insertion was chosen for the lower arch and the gold crowns were milled in the laboratory, allowing mesial proximal surfaces or guide planes parallel to the chosen path of insertion. In addition, mesio-occlusal rest seats, buccal ledges and lingual clasp grooves were incorporated within the gold casting (Figure 2.10.7). Tooth preparation involved supragingival chamfer margins extending beyond the cores into tooth structure. It is recommended that ledges or rest seat preparations should be made into the abutment preparations, to allow an adequate thickness of metal.

- The upper left canine was restored using a metal ceramic crown, with milled features on the metal occlusal and palatal surfaces to facilitate the upper RPD design (Figure 2.10.8).

- The upper denture was designed prior to tooth preparation and it was decided to include a significantly deep palatal ledge. This provides additional support and indirect retention to the removable prostheses. An added advantage of having a bracing component fitting into a prepared ledge in the crown is that it complements the contour of the tooth.

- Following construction of these milled crowns, the new restorations and chrome frameworks were trialled to ensure a precision fit at the chosen paths of insertion, and even contact at the increased occlusal vertical dimension. Once this had been confirmed, the cast restorations were cemented with a resin-modified glass ionomer cement.

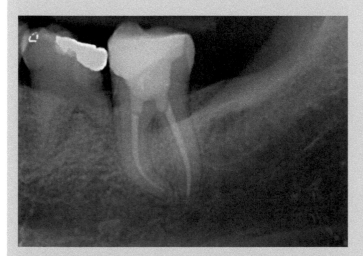

Figure 2.10.6 Root canal treatment completed on the lower second molar.

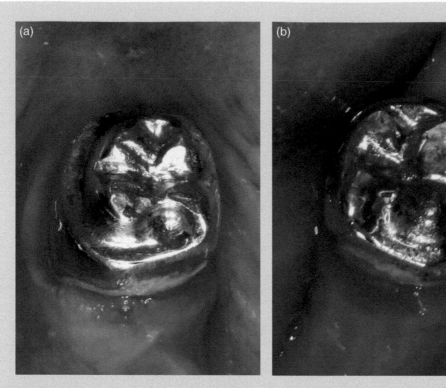

Figure 2.10.7 (a) and (b) Gold crowns fabricated with milled features for retention of the lower removable partial denture.

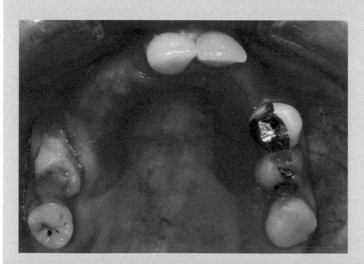

Figure 2.10.8 Upper arch with crowns fitted to aid denture retention.

- The design of the upper denture did not require any minor connectors to be placed on the upper central incisors. Therefore, it was decided to place new all-ceramic crowns on these teeth with distal guide planes. As these teeth had been prepared previously, only minimal adjustment and polishing of the preparations were required. Lithium disilicate glass-ceramic (IPS E.max,™ Ivoclar Vivadent,

Liechtenstein) was prescribed, as this has higher stress resistance than previous ceramics and achieves good aesthetics. Shade determination was undertaken, and this included a die shade determination using the IPS Natural Die Material Shade Guide (Ivoclar Vivadent, Liechtenstein). Once fabricated, the new crowns were trialled for shade, mould and marginal fit. The upper chrome framework was also trialled to ensure adequate fit at the chosen path of insertion. Following cleaning of the fitting surfaces, the restorations were cemented using a dual-cure translucent resin cement (Multilink Automix, Ivoclar Vivadent, Liechtenstein) (Figure 2.10.9).

- Although mobile, following discussion with the patient it was decided to restore the lower left lateral incisor and canine. A lingual plate was incorporated into the lower RPD, so that additions could be undertaken more easily should they require extraction in the future (Figure 2.10.10). It was ensured that the restorations had a minimum occlusal thickness of 2 mm, a dimension generally accepted for resin composite longevity in areas of occlusal loading.

- Appropriate oral and denture hygiene instruction was reinforced to the patient and a regular recall and maintenance schedule was organised. At her review appointment, the patient reported a high level of satisfaction with function and aesthetics (Figure 2.10.11).

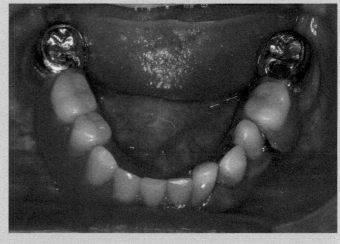

Figure 2.10.10 Lower denture inserted.

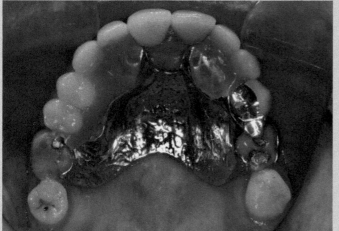

Figure 2.10.9 Upper denture inserted.

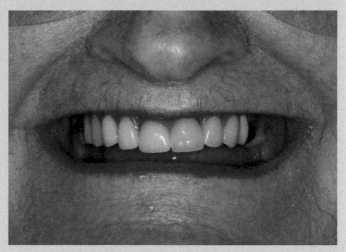

Figure 2.10.11 Final result at review.

Self-Study Questions

1. When designing a cobalt-chromium removable partial denture, what does support refer to?
   a. Resistance to displacement of the denture due to rotational forces on the saddle
   b. Resistance to displacement of the saddle away from the ridge
   c. Resistance to displacement of the saddle towards the ridge
   d. Resistance to horizontal forces exerted on abutment teeth when withdrawing clasps from undercuts
   e. Resistance to horizontal forces exerted on the saddle by the oral musculature

2. Which of the following are appropriate major connectors for a lower partial denture?
   a. Lingual plate
   b. Horseshoe
   c. Ring connector
   d. Lingual bar

3. Does provision of a cuspal coverage restoration have a positive impact on survival for endodontically treated posterior teeth?
   a. Yes
   b. No

Answers are located at the end of the case

Self-Study Answers

1. c. Resistance to displacement of the saddle towards the ridge[1]

2. a. Lingual plate and d. Lingual bar

3. a. Yes[3]

References

1 Owall B, Budtz-Jorgensen E, Davenport J, et al. (2002). Removable partial denture design: a need to focus on hygienic principles? *International Journal of Prosthodontics* 15: 371–378.

2 Studer P, Wettstein C, Lehner C, et al. (2001). Long-term survival estimates of cast gold inlays and onlays with their analysis of failure. *Journal of Oral Rehabilitation* 27: 461–472.

3 Ng YL, Mann V, Gulabivala K (2010). Tooth survival following non-surgical root canal treatment: a systematic review of the literature. *International Endodontic Journal* 43: 171–189.

Case 11

Utilising Upper and Lower Overdentures for a Partially Dentate Patient

With Contribution from Sayaka Tada

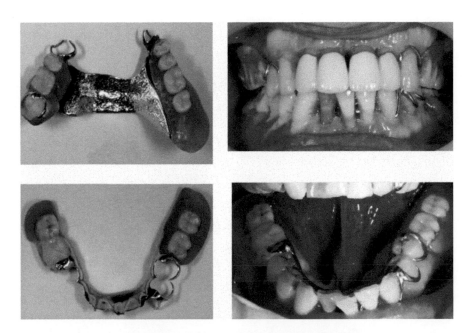

Figure 2.11.1 The patient at initial presentation, including his upper and lower partial dentures.

A. Case Story

A 72-year-old partially dentate male presented having difficulties wearing his upper and lower removable partial dentures (Figure 2.11.1). The patient had been wearing this set of dentures for a number of years and he was now experiencing significant difficulties with chewing. He was also unhappy with the appearance of his own remaining natural teeth and felt that a number of them were becoming increasingly mobile. The patient was an irregular dental attender and had not visited his dentist since the dentures were fitted three years ago. A full periodontal examination revealed a diagnosis of chronic generalised periodontal disease with Grade II and Grade III mobility. The treatment plan developed with the patient included extraction of hopeless teeth, with utilisation of some remaining teeth as overdenture abutments. Cast root caps were used, with new upper and lower dentures constructed.

LEARNING GOALS AND OBJECTIVES

- Appreciate that the use of natural overdenture abutments can significantly improve the retention of partial or complete removable prostheses
- Understand that natural tooth-retained overdentures often constitute the last resort before edentulism and may aid in this transition, especially in very old patients with reduced adaptive capacities
- Understand the need for correct design, preparation and aftercare for overdentures with cast copings, which can then provide a valid treatment option in partially dentate patients[1]

Case 13

Tooth Replacement According to the Principles of the Shortened Dental Arch

With Contribution from Conor McLister, Gerry McKenna and Haileigh McCarthy

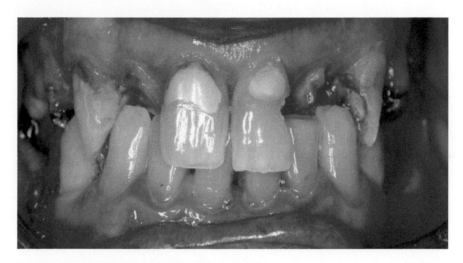

Figure 2.13.1 The patient's teeth at the initial consultation appointment.

A. Case Story

A 64-year-old male attended for dental treatment having neglected his teeth for a number of years. He was having pain from a number of broken teeth and had lost his upper partial denture. He had not attended a general dental practitioner for over five years, but was aware that his teeth were now 'in a bit of a state' (Figure 2.13.1). The patient was missing natural teeth in the upper and lower arches, but had never worn a lower removable prosthesis. He was aware that his oral hygiene had deteriorated significantly, but he was determined to address this. He was planning to attend his granddaughter's wedding in approximately 12 months' time and this was a motivating factor in seeking treatment.

LEARNING GOALS AND OBJECTIVES

- Understand that primary disease, notably dental caries in this case, must be controlled before considering more advanced treatment, including tooth replacement options; if patients are unable to maintain oral hygiene without a prosthesis in place, then this will be almost impossible once further restorations have been placed
- Understand that a variety of treatment planning strategies can be used when considering replacing missing teeth in older adults, including functionally orientated treatment such as the shortened dental arch (SDA) concept[1]
- Use of the SDA concept avoids the need for a removable partial denture (RPD) in one or both arches, while providing a functional, aesthetic dentition which is easier to maintain[2]

B. Medical History

- Rheumatoid arthritis affecting shoulders and legs – patient walks with the aid of a walking stick
- High blood pressure
- High cholesterol
- Under investigation for type II diabetes with his general medical practitioner

C. Dental History

- Patient presents with fractured and carious teeth including both upper lateral incisors
- Patient has been provided with an upper RPD, but this has been lost; patient did accommodate well to the RPD
- Patient is aware that he is missing posterior teeth in the lower arch, but has never worn a lower RPD
- Patient has not attended a general dental practitioner for approximately five years
- Patient is aware that his oral hygiene practices are currently substandard, but he is motivated to improve

D. Medications

- Valsartan (angiotensin II receptor antagonist) 80 mg once daily
- Rosuvastatin (CoA reductase inhibitor) 20 mg once daily
- Clopidogrel (anticoagulant) 75 mg once daily
- Ibuprofen topical gel (non-steroidal anti-inflammatory) as required
- Aspirin (non-steroidal anti-inflammatory) 150 mg daily

E. Social History

- Patient lives independently with his wife
- He is a retired postman and is socially active
- Smoking: approximately 5 cigarettes per day
- Alcohol: approximately 10 units of alcohol per week

F. Extraoral Examination

- Temporomandibular joint (TMJ): nothing abnormal detected, mouth opening normal
- Muscles of mastication: nothing abnormal detected
- Lymph nodes: nothing abnormal detected

G. Soft Tissue Examination

- No significant findings

H. Clinical Findings/Problem List

- Oral hygiene poor throughout the mouth
- Heavily restored dentition

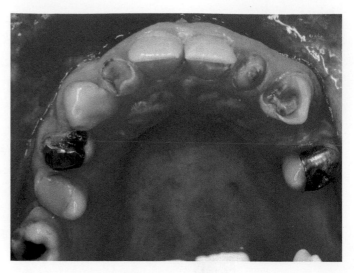

Figure 2.13.2 Upper teeth, including unrestorable upper lateral incisors.

- Caries/fractured teeth in upper arch; upper lateral incisors are grossly carious and unrestorable (Figures 2.13.2 and 2.13.3)
- Missing posterior units in upper and lower arches
- Patient would like to have a new upper RPD constructed, no history of wearing lower RPD
- Tooth charting:

		6	5	4	3	2	1	1	2	3		5			
	7			4	3	2	1	1	2	3	4				

- Basic periodontal examination:

2	1	–
1	2	–

I. Diagnoses

- Caries and fractured teeth
- Poor oral hygiene
- Partially dentate in upper and lower arches

CLINICAL DECISION MAKING – DETERMINING FACTORS

- The patient has neglected his natural dentition for a number of years and so initial treatment should be centred around pain relief, stabilisation and instituting an effective oral hygiene programme, before undertaking any complex treatment.
- A number of fractured and carious teeth in the upper arch were deemed unrestorable with large carious lesions extending subgingivally.[3] The unrestorable teeth were extracted under local anaesthesia, with other carious lesions restored using direct materials, including composite resin for coronal cavities (CeramX Universal™, Dentsply, USA) and glass ionomer for root surface cavities (Fuji IX GP Extra™, GC Corporation, Japan). Retained roots in the lower arch were also extracted.

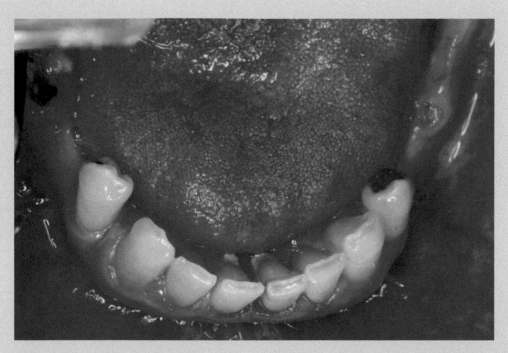

Figure 2.13.3 Lower teeth, including retained roots.

- Extensive oral hygiene instruction was provided and compliance monitored during the initial phase of treatment. High-fluoride toothpaste was prescribed for the patient (Duraphat® 5000 ppm Fluoride, Colgate-Palmolive, UK). Non-surgical periodontal treatment was carried out in all quadrants.
- After the initial phase of treatment, consideration was given to replacing missing teeth in the upper and lower arches. In the upper arch, the patient had multiple spaces and had previously accommodated well to an upper partial denture. He was keen to have a new removable prosthesis constructed as he was now missing upper anterior teeth. As the patient's oral condition was judged to be stable, a cobalt-chromium upper partial denture was pre-scribed after management of failing restorations and caries (Figure 2.13.4). This was designed by the clinician to provide a tooth-supported prosthesis which covered a small area of the hard palate and was clear of the gingival margins, thus facilitating maintenance of oral hygiene.[4]
- In the lower arch a number of treatment options were discussed with the patient, including a lower removable partial denture. The patient had retained lower anterior teeth, but without any lower poste-rior teeth. This pattern of tooth retention would have necessitated a lower Kennedy Class I bilateral

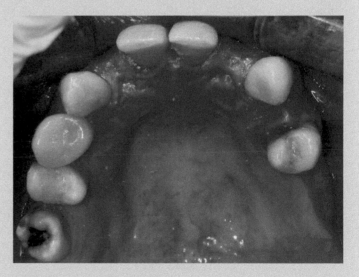

Figure 2.13.4 Upper arch after caries management, removal of unrestorable teeth and replacement of failing restorations.

free end saddle denture. Instead, the principles of the shortened dental arch (SDA) concept were utilised to provide the patient with a functional dentition of 10 occluding pairs using two adhesive resin-bonded bridges.[5]
- The SDA concept is very applicable to partially dentate older adults. Considerable evidence suggests that older patients prefer this functionally orientated treatment approach over RPDs. Evidence also shows that the SDA concept has a

positive impact on oral health-related quality of life, chewing ability and some aspects of nutrition.[6] Maintenance is considerably easier and provision of treatment is more cost effective than traditional RPDs.[7]

- Adhesive bridges can provide a simple and minimally invasive solution to replace missing teeth. Case selection is crucial and the amount of available enamel for bonding on the abutment teeth will ultimately govern success. A careful examination of the patient's static and dynamic occlusion is extremely important, as pontics provided should act as a light holding contact in intercuspal position (ICP) and not be involved in guidance movements.
- In this case, the amalgam restorations on the lower premolars were replaced with composite resin (CeramX Universal™, Dentsply, USA).
- Following the addition of silicone heavy and light body impressions, the laboratory was instructed to provide a rigid bridge framework made from nickel chromium,

a base metal alloy. Full palatal metal coverage was prescribed, with a minimum thickness of 0.7 mm providing sufficient resistance to dislodgement.

- A modified ridge lap porcelain fused to metal pontic was requested. Following trial of the restoration, the fitting metal surface was sandblasted chairside with 50 μm alumina to enhance retention. Cementation was undertaken with opaque resin cement (Panavia 21, Kuraray, Japan), which demonstrates prolonged high bond strengths and increases restoration longevity (Figure 2.13.5).
- The static and dynamic occlusion was rechecked using articulating paper to ensure that the planned occlusal scheme had been achieved.
- The patient was provided with a functional and aesthetic dentition which should be more easy to maintain than if an RPD had been provided. He has been reviewed at 6 and 12 months since treatment was completed and his oral hygiene has remained good (Figure 2.13.6).

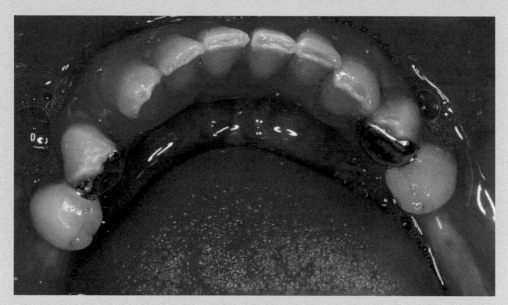

Figure 2.13.5 Adhesive bridges placed in lower arch to provide the patient with a functional dentition.

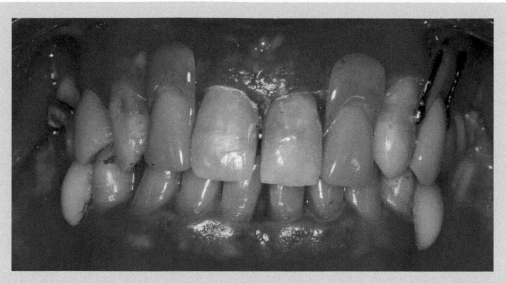

Figure 2.13.6 Final result incorporating upper removable partial denture and lower shortened dental arch.

Self-Study Questions

1. When designing a cobalt-chromium removable partial denture, which elements can provide direct retention?
    a. Major connector
    b. Minor connectors
    c. Saddles
    d. Clasps
    e. Rest seats

2. When writing a laboratory prescription for a resin-bonded bridge, which is the most common metal wing for the abutment?
    a. Chrome cobalt at least 0.7 mm thick
    b. Chrome cobalt at least 1.0 mm thick
    c. Nickel chromium at least 0.7 mm thick
    d. Nickel chromium at least 1.0 mm thick
    e. Titanium at least 1.0 mm thick

Answers are located at the end of the case

Self-Study Answers

1. d. Clasps

2. c. Nickel chromium at least 0.7 mm thick[4]

References

1 McKenna G, Allen PF, O'Mahony D, et al. (2015). The impact of rehabilitation using removable partial dentures and functionally orientated treatment on oral health-related quality of life: a randomized controlled clinical trial. *Journal of Dentistry* 43: 66–71.

2 Jepson NJ, Moynihan PJ, Kelly PJ, et al. (2001). Caries incidence following restoration of shortened lower dental arches in a randomized controlled trial. *British Dental Journal* 191: 140–144.

3 Quilligan G, McKenna G, Allen PF (2016). The restorability assessment and endodontic access cavity interface. *Dental Update* 43: 933–938.

4 Allen PF, McKenna G, Creugers N (2011). Prosthodontic care for elderly patients. *Dental Update* 38: 460–470.

5 Käyser A. (1981). Shortened dental arches and oral function. *Journal of Oral Rehabilitation* 8: 457–462.

6 Wallace S, Samietz S, Abbas M, et al. (2018). Impact of prosthodontic rehabilitation on the masticatory performance of partially dentate older patients: can it predict nutritional state? Results from an RCT. *Journal of Dentistry* 68: 66–71.

7 McKenna G, Allen PF, Woods N, et al. (2014). Cost-effectiveness of tooth replacement strategies for partially dentate elderly: a randomised controlled clinical trial. *Community Dentistry and Oral Epidemiology* 42: 366–374.

Case 14

Use of a Natural Pontic to Replace a Lower Incisor Lost Due to Periodontal Disease

With Contribution from Celeste van Heumen, Gerry McKenna and Brian Rosenberg

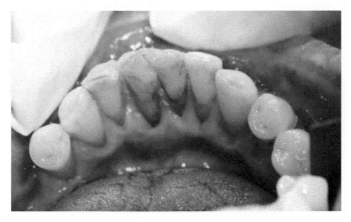

Figure 2.14.1 Lower incisor teeth at initial presentation.

A. Case story

A 73-year-old female was undergoing treatment for periodontal disease. The patient had previously been a smoker and had been receiving non-surgical periodontal treatment (NSPT) for her lower natural teeth at regular intervals for a number of years. The patient had a number of mobile teeth in the lower arch, but the lower right central incisor was becoming increasingly mobile and causing discomfort (Figure 2.14.1). The patient was informed that this tooth had a very poor long-term prognosis. Despite further periodontal treatment, the tooth remained symptomatic and the patient requested that it be removed. A number of treatment options were discussed with the patient for replacing the lower incisor, including a removable partial denture. While the patient wore a full upper denture, she did not have any experience of wearing a lower prosthesis and was reluctant to consider this option. Instead of an immediate lower denture, it was decided to utilise the extracted tooth as a natural pontic and thus maintain a function dentition in the lower arch.

LEARNING GOALS AND OBJECTIVES

- Appreciate that while NSPT can be used effectively to manage and maintain periodontal disease in older adults, some teeth will not respond successfully
- Recognise that in patients with periodontally involved teeth, it may be advisable to avoid a removable partial denture as this can further complicate plaque control and periodontal maintenance, particularly if constructed in acrylic resin; a definitive fixed prosthesis is not recommended immediately following an extraction, as hard and soft tissue remodelling will occur under the pontic, leaving a stagnation area and an unaesthetic appearance
- Understand that a natural pontic can be used as a short- to medium-term option to replace a missing tooth immediately after extraction; it is vitally important that the occlusion is checked and adjusted, as excessive loading or involvement in guidance movements will result in the natural pontic being lost very quickly.

B. Medical History

- Hypertension
- Osteoarthritis
- Previous treatment for breast cancer
- Asthma
- Mild depression

C. Dental History

- Patient is edentate in the upper arch and has worn a full upper prosthesis successfully for over 30 years
- Lower anterior teeth retained, but long history of chronic periodontal disease
- Upper teeth and lower posterior teeth lost due to periodontal disease

Self-Study Questions

1. How would implant survival rates for older adults be expected to compare to younger patients?
   a. Higher
   b. Lower
   c. Comparable

2. Which of the following is an advantage of screw-retained implant prostheses?
   a. Retrievability
   b. Improved aesthetics
   c. Lower laboratory costs
   d. Increased patient acceptance

3. Which of the following systemic conditions/treatments would contraindicate dental implant treatment for an older patient?
   a. High-dose intravenous antiresorptive therapy (ART)
   b. Liver cirrhosis
   c. Xerostomia
   d. Cardiovascular disease

Answers are located at the end of the case

Self-Study Answers

1. c. Comparable[5]

2. a. Retrievability

3. a. High-dose intravenous antiresorptive therapy (ART)[5]

References

1 Sarita PTN, Kreulen CM, Witter DJ, Creugers NHJ (2003). Signs and symptoms of temporo-mandibular dysfunction in adults with shortened dental arches in Tanzania. *International Journal of Prosthodontics* 16: 265–270.

2 Witter DJ, Creugers NHJ, Kreulen CM, de Haan AFJ (2001). Occlusal stability in shortened dental arches. *Journal of Dental Research* 80: 432–436.

3 Witter DJ, Van Palenstein-Helderman WH, Käyser AF, Creugers NHJ (1999). The shortened dental arch concept and its implications on oral health care. *Community Dentistry and Oral Epidemiology* 22: 249–258.

4 Creugers NHJ, Witter DJ, van 't Spijker A, et al. (2010). Occlusion and temporomandibular function among subjects with shortened dental arches with mandibular bilateral distal extension removable partial dentures. *International Journal of Dentistry Article ID* 807850.

5 Schimmel M, Srinivasan M, McKenna G, Müller F (2018). Effect of advanced age and/or systemic medical conditions on dental implant survival: a systematic review and meta-analysis. *Clinical Oral Implants Research* 29: 311–330.

6 Gerritsen AE, Witter DJ, Bronkhorst EM, Creugers NHJ (2013). An observational cohort study on shortened dental arches – clinical course during a period of 27–35 years. *Clinical Oral Investigations* 17: 859–866.

7 Zhang Q, Witter DJ, Bronkhorst EM, et al. (2014). Occlusal tooth wear in Chinese adults with shortened dental arches. *Journal of Oral Rehabilitation* 41: 101–107.

Chapter 3

Management of Failing Restorations

Case 16

Endodontic Treatment for a Fractured Tooth and Conversion to an Overdenture Abutment

With Contribution from Graham Quilligan

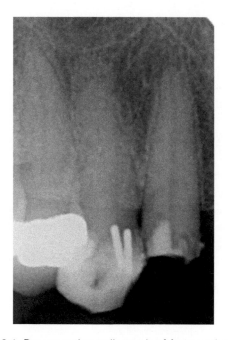

Figure 3.16.1 Pre-operative radiograph of fractured canine.

A. Case Story

An 81-year-old female who has been receiving intravenous bisphosphonate injections for seven years presented with a fractured maxillary right canine. The tooth had previously been heavily restored with a number of different composite restorations. After an initial clinical examination, it was determined that the tooth was not predictably restorable with a direct or indirect restoration as a ferrule could not be provided (Figure 3.16.1). Crown lengthening was not considered, as this surgical manipulation of the mucosa and alveolar bone could lead to bisphosphonate-related osteonecrosis of the jaws (BRONJ).[1] When the risks of BRONJ following extraction were discussed with the patient, she was very keen to avoid extraction. She wished to have the tooth treated endodontically and retained. The plan was to retain the tooth as support for an

overdenture. Root canal treatment was undertaken under rubber dam isolation and the tooth restored with amalgam to provide a coronal seal. The tooth was added to her current maxillary denture following endodontic treatment.

LEARNING GOALS AND OBJECTIVES

- Appreciate that determining the restorability of a tooth and planning for the final restoration are crucially important before undertaking endodontic treatment[2]
- Appreciate that where a fractured tooth is adjacent to a removable prosthesis, consideration should be given to utilisation as an overdenture abutment to allow the patient to retain their tooth and increase the support for the denture[3]
- Recognise that large numbers of older patients are prescribed bisphosphonates for a variety of medical conditions, including osteoporosis, Paget's disease of bone, and bone metastases[4]
- Understand that patients taking bisphosphonates are at risk of developing BRONJ after extractions, particularly when they are administered intravenously[1]
- Identify fractured teeth that can be retained as overdenture abutments following root canal treatment

B. Medical History

- Hypertension
- Osteoporosis
- Rheumatoid arthritis
- High cholesterol controlled by medication and dietary advice
- Allergy to penicillin

C. Dental History

- Partially dentate and wearing an upper acrylic partial denture
- Heavily restored dentition with a large number of direct and indirect restorations
- Symptomatic attender, last visited over 12 months previously

D. Medications

- Aspirin (non-steroidal anti-inflammatory) 150 mg daily
- Simvastatin (CoA reductase inhibitor) 40 mg once daily
- Atenolol (beta blocker) 50 mg twice per day
- Zoledronic acid (intravenous bisphosphonate) 4 mg every 4 weeks

E. Social History

- Widowed, independently living
- Socially active
- Non-smoker
- Drinks eight units of alcohol per week (wine)

F. Extraoral Examination

- Temporomandibular joint (TMJ): nothing abnormal detected
- Muscles of mastication: nothing abnormal detected
- Lymph nodes: nothing abnormal detected

G. Soft Tissue Examination

- No significant findings

H. Clinical Findings/Problem List

- Partially dentate and wearing an upper acrylic partial denture
- Fractured upper right canine, sensitive to cold air and slightly tender to percussion
- Heavily restored dentition
- Tooth charting:

	6	5	4	3		1					6	7
	6			3	2	1	1	2	3		5	

- Basic periodontal examination:

1	2	1
–	2	–

I. Diagnoses

- Partially dentate upper and lower arches
- Fractured 13 at gingival margin, caries 13
- Unrestorable 13 due to lack of coronal tooth structure and ferrule

---

CLINICAL DECISION MAKING – DETERMINING FACTORS

- The fractured tooth was not suitable for a predictable extracoronal restoration due to the limited amount of natural tooth tissue remaining supragingivally. Given the small amount of remaining coronal tooth tissue, a cast post and core would have been required to support a crown. There was insufficient natural tooth tissue for a ferrule that could support a cast post and core crown. A direct fibre post was also not suitable due to the lack of coronal tooth tissue.
- Extraction was best avoided in this case due to the patient taking oral bisphosphonates for prevention of osteoporosis (BRONJ).[1]
- The patient was already wearing a upper acrylic partial denture, which she was managing well. It was decided that the canine could be treated endodontically and utilised as an overdenture abutment. The existing denture could be modified simply and an acrylic tooth added to fill the space. Canine teeth are regarded as good choices for an overdenture abutment as they have long straight roots and are located anteriorly.
- Rubber dam was placed and the endodontic procedure was completed in one appointment with rotary files (Protaper Universal, Dentsply Sirona, USA). Sodium hypochlorite was used as an irrigant to sterilise the root canal system. The canal was obturated using gutta percha and a calcium hydroxide root canal sealer (Sealapex™, Kerr Dental, USA) (Figure 3.16.2).
- A direct final restoration in dental amalgam was placed to provide a coronal seal (Figure 3.16.3).
- An impression was taken of the partial denture in situ using alginate and sent to the dental laboratory for an addition of the canine. The partial denture was relined and the overdenture abutment utilised to support the denture. The partial denture was returned to the patient and fitted three hours later.

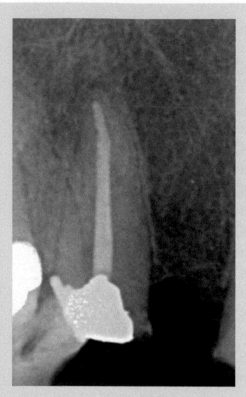

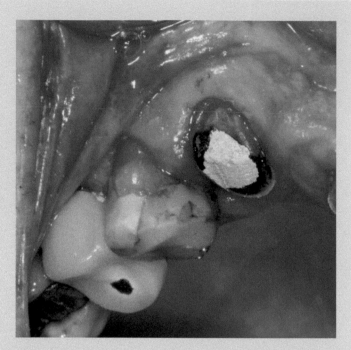

Figure 3.16.3 Post-operative clinical scenario with amalgam restoration in situ.

Figure 3.16.2 Post-obturation radiograph.

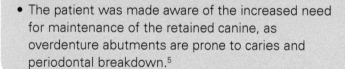

- The patient was made aware of the increased need for maintenance of the retained canine, as overdenture abutments are prone to caries and periodontal breakdown.[5]

- Fluoride varnish (Duraphat varnish 22,600 ppm fluoride, Colgate, USA) was painted onto the overdenture abutment at each maintenance visit.

Self-Study Questions

1. What is the reported half-life of alendronate in bone?
   a. 12 months
   b. 3 years
   c. 10 years
   d. 90 days

2. Is it recommended to advise patients prescribed bisphosphonates to take a drug holiday immediately before an invasive dental procedure to reduce the risk of BRONJ?
   a. Yes
   b. No

3. Which of the following statements about overdenture abutments is incorrect?
   a. They are at increased risk of developing caries
   b. They are plaque retentive
   c. They may require elective endodontic treatment
   d. They reduce the risk of denture fracture
   e. They should be located symmetrically in the arch

Answers are located at the end of the case

Self-Study Answers

1. c. 10 years[1]

2. b. No[1]

3. d. They reduce the risk of denture fracture

References

1 Scottish Dental Clinical Effectiveness Programme (2017). *Oral Health Management of Patients at Risk of Medication-related Osteonecrosis of the Jaw*. NHS Education for Scotland, Edinburgh.

2 Quilligan G, McKenna G, Allen PF (2016). The restorability assessment and endodontic access cavity interface. *Dental Update* 43: 933–938.

3 Allen PF, McKenna G, Creugers N (2011). Prosthodontic care for elderly patients. *Dental Update* 38: 460–470.

4 Ghezzi EM, Ship JA (2000). Systemic diseases and their treatments in the elderly: impact on oral health. *Journal of Public Health Dentistry* 60: 289–296.

5 Mercouriadis-Howald A, Rollier N, Tada S, et al. (2018). Loss of natural abutment teeth with cast copings retaining over-dentures: a systematic review and meta-analysis. *Journal of Prosthodontic Research* 62: 407–415.

Case 17

Managing the Failing Restored Dentition: Replacement of Failing Crowns

With Contribution from Graham Quilligan

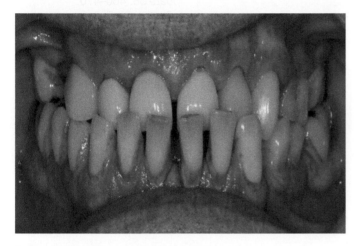

Figure 3.17.1 Pre-treatment anterior view.

A. Case Story

A 69-year-old male attended with a chief complaint of 'rough edges to his tongue from the crowns on his front teeth'. He had crowns placed on his maxillary anterior teeth approximately 10 years previously. The patient presented with a Class III incisal relationship, but he had no concerns about the aesthetics associated with this (Figure 3.17.1). He had always had a reverse overjet and admitted that this was a familial trait. He did not have any functional concerns and found that he could eat and chew a wide variety of foods.

LEARNING GOALS AND OBJECTIVES

- Recognise that when dismantling or removing existing fixed prosthodontics, it is vitally important to undertake a careful restorability assessment before undertaking further treatment[1]; where teeth are unrestorable, this should be identified as early as possible and further treatment planning developed to cope with their loss

- Appreciate that care needs to be taken when removing old indirect restorations in potentially fragile teeth; crowns and bridges should be sectioned and prized off rather than using an aggressive crown and bridge remover, which could fracture the core
- Understand that tooth preparations for indirect restorations need to be guided by the materials chosen for the final restorations; clinicians should work closely with their technical colleagues to ensure that adequate space is created for the restorative materials prescribed

B. Medical History
- Hypertension
- Osteoarthritis
- Well-controlled type II diabetes mellitus
- Angina

C. Dental History
- Regular dental attender, attending practice dental hygienist for six-monthly non-surgical periodontal treatment
- Previous extractions, fillings, root canal treatments and full-coverage crowns
- No dental anxiety reported

D. Medications
- Bendroflumethiazide (diuretic) 5 mg daily
- Aspirin (non-steroidal anti-inflammatory) 75 mg daily
- Ibuprofen gel (non-steroidal anti-inflammatory) as required
- Metformin hydrochloride (anti-hyperglycaemic) 500 mg daily
- Glyceryl trinitrate spray (nitrate) 400 mg as required

Self-Study Questions

1. Which retrograde endodontic filling material promotes optimum healing?
   a. Composite
   b. Glass ionomer cement
   c. Mineral trioxide aggregate (MTA)
   d. Amalgam

2. What is the most conservative way to remove a bridge?
   a. Placing a very sticky material between the teeth
   b. Sectioning the bridge
   c. Tapping the bridge off
   d. Using a forceps to loosen each abutment

3. Which material should be used to construct an immediate partial denture?
   a. Cobalt-chromium
   b. Acrylic resin
   c. Stainless steel

Answers are located at the end of the case

Self-Study Answers

1. c. Mineral trioxide aggregate (MTA)[3]

2. b. Sectioning the bridge

3. b. Acrylic resin

References

1 Quilligan G, McKenna G, Allen PF (2016). The restorability assessment and endodontic access cavity interface. *Dental Update* 43: 933–938.

2 Brocklehurst PR, McKenna G, Schimmel M, et al. (2018). How do we incorporate patient views into the design of healthcare services for older people: a discussion paper. *BMC Oral Health* 18: 61.

3 Apaydin ES, Shabahang S, Torebinejad M (2004). Hard-tissue healing after application of fresh or set MTA as root-end-filling material. *Journal of Endodontics* 30: 21–24.

Case 19

Dismantling a Long-Span Fixed Bridge and Replacement with a Removable Partial Denture

With Contribution from Gerry McKenna and Finbarr Allen

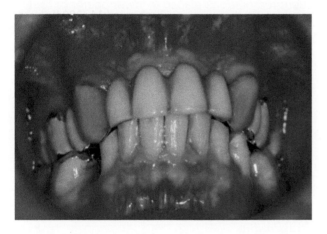

Figure 3.19.1 Patient at initial presentation; note the poor aesthetics of the existing long-span fixed bridge.

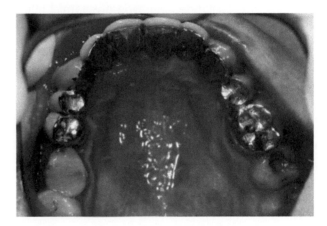

Figure 3.19.2 Palatal view demonstrating the extensive nature of the existing bridge.

A. Case Story

A 64-year-old male presented with a failing extensive fixed bridge in the upper arch. The bridge had been placed over 15 years ago while the patient was in the army and serving overseas. He had not attended for regular maintenance of his dentition, but had recently registered with a general dental practitioner. While some conservative and periodontal treatment had recently been completed, issues had been noted with the bridge. It was loose and the patient was unhappy with the aesthetics (Figures 3.19.1 and 3.19.2). Clinical examination revealed caries on a number of abutment teeth. Several treatment options were discussed with the patient, including the use of dental implants, but he declined this for financial reasons. The patient was informed that a replacement bridge was not a viable treatment option given the number of teeth that were missing.

LEARNING GOALS AND OBJECTIVES

- Appreciate that long-span fixed prosthodontics are ill-advised for any age group; maintenance is

extremely challenging for the patient and failure can be catastrophic
- Understand that patient involvement in the treatment planning process is vitally important; particularly when a significant change is planned, for example a transition from fixed to removable prosthodontics, it is essential that the patent is involved in decision making and understands the rationale for clinical choices[1]
- Recognise that appropriately planned fixed prosthodontics can significantly aid in the retention of a removable prosthesis; it is important that the removable partial denture (RPD) is designed first with crowns, then constructed to facilitate the design

B. Medical History

- Irregular heart beat
- Type II diabetes mellitus
- Occasional angina

C. Dental History

- Large amount of dental work completed approximately 15 years ago while in the army
- Anterior maxillary teeth lost due to caries
- Heavily restored dentition, including a long-span conventional bridge in the upper arch
- Patient currently registered with a general dental practitioner, but has been an irregular attender over the last 5 years

D. Medications

- Clopidogrel (anticoagulant) 75 mg once daily
- Metformin hydrochloride (anti-hyperglycaemic) 500 mg daily
- Glyceryl trinitrate spray (nitrate) 400 mg as required
- No known drug allergies

E. Social History

- Retired army officer
- Lives with wife
- Provides child care for grandchildren
- Current smoker (3–4 cigarettes per day)
- Alcohol use: 20 units per week

F. Extraoral Examination

- Temporomandibular joint (TMJ): asymptomatic click on left side opening
- Muscles of mastication: nothing abnormal detected
- Lymph nodes: nothing abnormal detected

G. Soft Tissue Examination

- No significant findings

H. Clinical Findings/Problem List

- Long-span conventional bridge in upper arch retained with three abutment teeth: 13, 16 and 23
- Aesthetics of conventional bridge very poor, appears to have different shades of porcelain on anterior and posterior teeth
- Caries in abutment teeth
- Bridge loose but not easily removed
- Recent restorations placed in lower posterior teeth
- Temporary restoration in 26
- Oral hygiene fair
- Tooth charting:

8	7	6		3				3		6	7
	7	6		3	2	1	1	2	3	4	6

- Basic periodontal examination:

1	2	1
2	2	2

I. Diagnoses

- Failing conventional bridge in maxilla
- Temporary restoration 26

CLINICAL DECISION MAKING – DETERMINING FACTORS

- The current conventional bridge is failing: the bridge is loose with caries in the abutment teeth. The aesthetics of the bridge are poor: the shade of the porcelain on the anterior teeth appears to be different to the posterior teeth.
  Oral hygiene is fair, but food is packing under the conventional bridge; patient admits it is very challenging to maintain.
- A number of treatment options were discussed with the patient, including provision of a new conventional bridge, use of implant-retained bridgework and an Removable Partial Denture (RPD).
- The patient was informed that clinical decision making would have to be finalised after the bridge had been removed and the underlying abutments assessed. The clinical assessment included vitality testing and assessment of restorability.[2] It was determined that the abutment teeth 13, 16 and 23

were vital and restorable. The clinical decision was also made to consider a crown on 26, as this tooth was heavily restored.
- The patient was very keen to consider a new conventional bridge, but this was advised against given the condition of the abutment teeth and the numbers of missing teeth to be replaced. The patient was informed that in order to provide a fixed prosthodontic solution, dental implants would need to be utilised.
- For financial reasons the patient did not wish to consider dental implants. Therefore further assessment of available bone volume and implant planning was not undertaken.
- A treatment plan was developed that included:
- Removal of the existing bridge
  o Provision of an immediate upper acrylic RPD
  o Utilisation of the bridge abutments as abutments for the RPD

o Provision of crowns on the abutment teeth with features to facilitate a definitive cobalt-chromium framework RPD

- In order to provide the upper RPD in combination with milled crowns with features, the denture design was completed first. Study models were made, mounted and surveyed to facilitate the denture design. In keeping with fundamental principles of removable prosthodontics, a path of insertion was chosen that differed from the path of natural displacement.[3]

- Crown preparations were undertaken in keeping with the denture design. A polyvinyl siloxane (PVS) impression was taken in a spaced and perforated special tray with adhesive. A single impression was taken of the whole upper arch so that the dental laboratory could manufacture both the crowns and the denture framework on the same master model. An extremely accurate impression is required for this technique. Alternatively, the crowns and denture framework can be constructed separately, but this does require more clinical visits.

- Porcelain fused to metal crowns were constructed with metal positioned where the denture framework would contact the crowns on 13, 16, 23 and 26 (Figure 3.19.3). As the crowns and metal framework were constructed together, they were tried into the patient's mouth together. As the fit of all components was judged to be satisfactory, denture construction continued through the usual stages of jaw registration, wax try-in and fit.

- At the final appointment, the crowns were cemented using glass ionomer cement

(FujiCem, GC Corporation, Japan), with the denture inserted immediately after seating. This ensured that both the fixed and removable components fitted extremely well together (Figure 3.19.4).

- The patient was extremely pleased with the final result (Figure 3.19.5). The comfort and retention of the metal framework denture helped to dispel his earlier reluctance to consider a removable prosthesis.

- The patient was reviewed 6 and 12 months after the denture was fitted and then he was discharged to his general dental practitioner for maintenance.

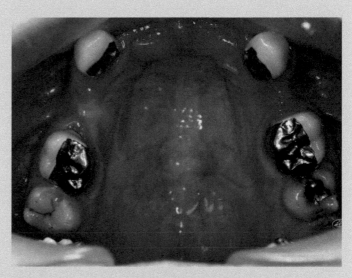

Figure 3.19.3 Crowns constructed to facilitate the design for the upper removable partial denture: note the mesial rests in 16 and 26 and the palatal features in 13 and 23.

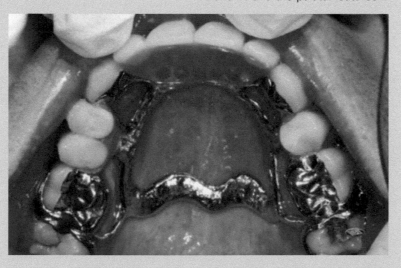

Figure 3.19.4 Fit of upper removable partial denture with components engaging in features on crowns on abutment teeth.

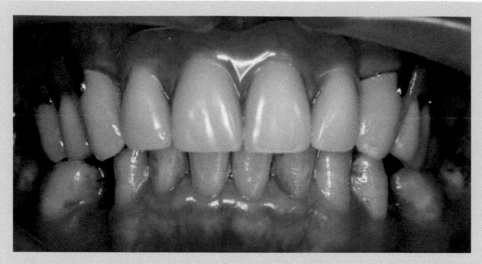

Figure 3.19.5 Final result 6 months after fit.

Self-Study Questions

1. What is surveying?
   a. A method of representing the movements of the temporomandibular joints
   b. A technique for fabricating and testing fixed and removable prostheses
   c. The procedure of locating the contour and position of the abutment teeth and associated structures after constructing an RPD
   d. The procedure of locating the contour and position of the abutment teeth and associated structures before designing an RPD
   e. The procedure used to ensure the creation of adequate interocclusal space during the preparation for a fixed prosthesis

2. Why are cobalt-chromium framework RPDs favoured over acrylic RPDs in older patients?
   a. Improved aesthetics
   b. Minimal gingival coverage that simplifies maintenance[3]
   c. Improved retention[3]
   d. Easier to provide additions

3. When providing an RPD in combination with crowns, which element should be designed first?
   a. Crowns
   b. RPD

Answers are located at the end of the case

Self-Study Answers

1. d. The procedure of locating the contour and position of the abutment teeth and associated structures before designing an RPD

2. b. Minimal gingival coverage that simplifies maintenance and c. Improved retention[3]
3. RPD

References

1 Brocklehurst PR, McKenna G, Schimmel M, et al. (2018). How do we incorporate patient views into the design of healthcare services for older people: a discussion paper. *BMC Oral Health* 18: 61.

2 Quilligan G, McKenna G, Allen PF (2016). The restorability assessment and endodontic access cavity interface. *Dental Update* 43: 933–938.

3 Allen PF, McKenna G, Creugers N (2011). Prosthodontic care for elderly patients. *Dental Update* 38: 460–470.

Case 20

Replacement of a Failing Implant Bridge for a Patient with Missing Lower Teeth

With Contribution from Nicola Holland, Gerry McKenna, Ciaran Moore and Robert Thompson

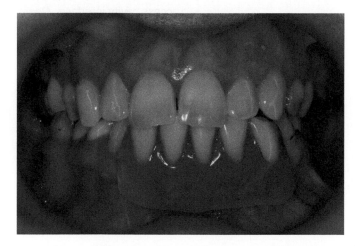

Figure 3.20.1 Patient at initial presentation; note the poor aesthetics of the acrylic flange and the wear on the prosthetic teeth.

A. Case Story

A 68-year-old female had received dental implant treatment approximately 15 years previously. She had been in a road traffic accident and had lost a number of teeth, most notably her lower incisors. She had been provided with an implant-retained bridge supported by two implants. A third implant had been placed at the time of surgery, but this had not been utilised due to poor positioning. The implants had been restored with a screw-retained bridge constructed using acrylic. The patient was in a yearly maintenance programme that included removal of the bridge periodically and cleaning. However, the bridge was now starting to deteriorate and part of the anterior acrylic flange had fractured, causing an ulcer (Figure 3.20.1). The patient was finding it more and more difficult to clean around the bridge and was experiencing increasing amounts of food packing underneath the bridge. A decision was made to replace the bridge to facilitate improved oral hygiene and better aesthetics.

LEARNING GOALS AND OBJECTIVES

- Understand that implant restorations have a finite lifespan and will need to be replaced periodically[1]
- Recognise that screw-retained prostheses will facilitate maintenance as well as repair and replacement better than cemented prostheses[2]
- Understand that where a significant amount of alveolar bone and soft tissues have been lost, pink acrylic or porcelain can be used to mask the defect
- Appreciate that it is vitally important that any implant prosthesis provided is cleansable for the patient and that an appropriate maintenance regime is developed

B. Medical History

- Hypertension
- Type II diabetes (well controlled with diet)
- Atrial fibrillation
- Asthma
- Early signs of osteoarthritis

C. Dental History

- Teeth previously lost due to trauma (road traffic accident)
- Heavily restored posterior teeth
- Implant-retained bridge provided approximately 15 years previously
- Regular attender with hygienist in general dental practice and yearly review in dental hospital where implant bridge was provided
- Implant bridge removed and cleaned once per year

D. Medications

- Clopidogrel (anticoagulant) 75 mg once daily
- Atorvastatin (CoA reductase inhibitor) 10 mg once daily
- Diazepam (benzodiazepine) 10 mg once daily

- Salbutamol (bronchodilator) 100 µg, up to four times daily
- Diclofenac (non-steroidal anti-inflammatory) 75 mg twice daily
- No known drug allergies

E.   Social History

- Widowed with grown-up children
- Lives alone
- Working as part-time office administrator
- No history of smoking
- Alcohol use: one bottle of wine per week

F.   Extraoral Examination

- Temporomandibular joint (TMJ): nothing abnormal detected
- Muscles of mastication: nothing abnormal detected
- Lymph nodes: nothing abnormal detected

G.   Soft Tissue Examination

- No significant findings

H.   Clinical Findings/Problem List

- Patient partially dentate in upper and lower arches; unrestored spaces are not a concern to her

- Oral hygiene good
- Implant-retained bridge replacing lower anterior teeth, constructed from acrylic and prosthetic teeth and showing signs of wear; large acrylic flange on bridge with small fracture on labial aspect; plaque deposits trapped under bridge
- Radiographic examination revealed no evidence of peri-implantitis or significant marginal bone loss associated with implants in lower anterior region
- Tooth charting:

		6	5	4	3	2	1	1	2	3	4	5		7	
		6	5	4	3						4	5			

- Basic periodontal examination:

1	1	1
1	–	1

I.   Diagnosis

- Failing implant-retained bridge in anterior mandible

CLINICAL DECISION MAKING – DETERMINING FACTORS

- Oral hygiene is good throughout the patient's mouth and she is actively maintaining the implant bridge, but this is increasingly challenging.
- The implant bridge is no longer serviceable and aesthetics could be improved with a new fixed prosthesis.
- Implant bridge is screw retained, which makes removal simple.
- Implants in situ are Regular Platform (RP) Branemark System (Nobel Biocare Services AG™, Switzerland). Clinical and radiographic assessments reveal no evidence of significant marginal bone loss or soft tissue inflammation. Food packing is clearly apparent on clinical examination and after removal of the bridge.
- An implant-level impression was taken in polyvinylsiloxane (PVS; Flexitime® Heavy Tray VPS Impression Solutions, Kulzer, Germany) using an open tray technique. Impression copings (5 mm Open Tray Branemark System RP) were attached to the implants (Figure 3.20.2).

- A jaw registration was performed using PVS (Blu-Mousse VPS Registration Material, Parkell, USA) and a bridge try-in created in wax with acrylic denture teeth (Figure 3.20.3).
- After consultation with the patient and the laboratory technician, the bridge was finished and fitted. Pink porcelain was used to compensate for the large vertical bone discrepancy in the anterior mandible. The final bridge was screw retained and the access holes were filled with composite (Figures 3.20.4 and 3.20.5).
- Considerations: appropriate three-dimensional positioning of the implants allowed for construction of a screw-retained bridge in this case. A screw-retained prosthesis allows for retrievability and can facilitate appropriate maintenance.[2] With a screw-retained prosthesis there is no requirement for cement to secure the bridge. In this case the patient had a large vertical bone discrepancy in the anterior mandible as a result of previous trauma. This area was managed using pink porcelain to provide an acceptable aesthetic result.

Care was taken to ensure that the final bridge with the pink porcelain in place was cleansable and easy to maintain for the patient. This was done with careful communication with the dental laboratory manufacturing the implant bridge.

- The patient is now once again on a careful maintenance routine that includes regular attendance with a hygienist in general dental practice and yearly review in the dental hospital.

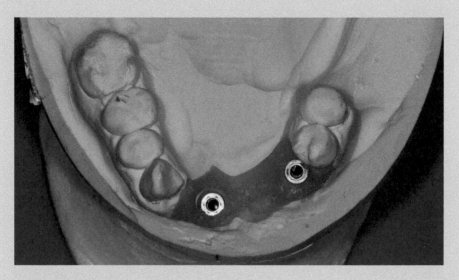

Figure 3.20.2 Working model created after implant-level impression.

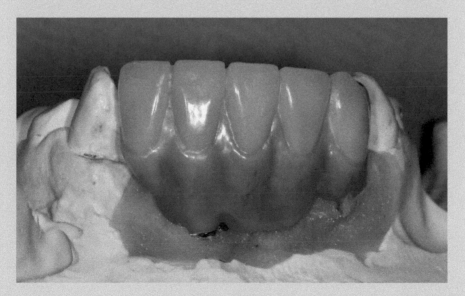

Figure 3.20.3 Wax try-in of new bridge.

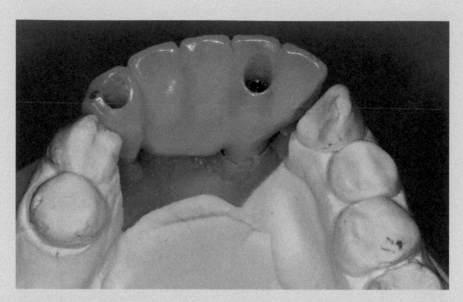

Figure 3.20.4 Bridge on working model prior to fit.

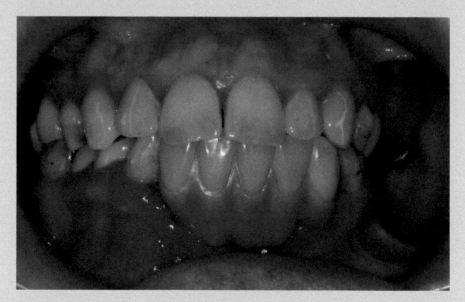

Figure 3.20.5 Final result after bridge fit.

Self-Study Questions

1. Which of the following techniques cannot be used to help plan the three-dimensional position of a dental implant?
   a. Diagnostic wax-up of the final restoration
   b. Construction of a surgical stent
   c. Virtual planning with cone beam CT scanning
   d. Clinical photography

2. Which material is most suitable to seal the screw access holes on a screw-retained implant prosthesis?
   a. Glass ionomer cement
   b. Composite resin
   c. Amalgam
   d. Mineral trioxide aggregate (MTA)

Self-Study Answers

1. a. Clinical photography

2. b. Composite resin

References

1 Pjetursson BE, Bragger U, Lang NP, Zwahlen M (2007). Comparison of survival and complication rates of tooth-supported fixed dental prostheses (FDPs) and implant-supported FDPs and single crowns (SCs). *Clinical Oral Implants Research* 18: 97–113.

2 Ma S, Fenton A (2015). Screw versus cement-retained implant prostheses: a systematic review of prosthodontic maintenance and complications. *International Journal of Prosthodontics* 28: 127–145.

Chapter 4

Management of Malignancy and Other Oral Conditions

Clinical Cases in Gerodontology, First Edition. Edited by Gerry McKenna, Finbarr Allen, and Francis Burke.
© 2021 John Wiley & Sons Ltd. Published 2021 by John Wiley & Sons Ltd.

- Tooth charting:

					3	2		1	2	3	4				
7	6	5	4	3	2	1	1	2	3	4	5				

- Basic periodontal examination:

–	2	–
3	2	2

I. Diagnoses

- Partially dentate in upper and lower arches
- Generalised severe non-carious tooth surface loss
- Caries and failing restorations
- Lack of posterior support and no reproducible ICP
- Chronic apical periodontitis associated with multiple lower anterior teeth

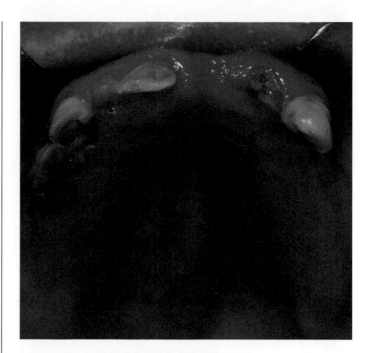

Figure 4.22.3 Pre-operative mandibular view.

CLINICAL DECISION MAKING – DETERMINING FACTORS

- The objective of the treatment was to eliminate the irritation to the patient's tongue and improve his oral function by replacing his missing teeth.
- On the advice of the patient's oncologist, extraction of teeth was to be avoided where possible due to the history of high-dose radiotherapy and previous ONJ.
- Unfortunately, the retained roots in the 46 region were not restorable and needed to be extracted atraumatically. The roots had associated periapical pathology, but were not amenable to endodontic treatment as there was insufficient tooth tissue to retain a rubber dam clamp.[3] It was decided that all other roots in the mandible would be retained as overdenture abutments and root canal treatment carried out where necessary.
- It was important to protect the remaining roots from further decay. The patient was at high risk of caries given his post-radiotherapy xerostomia.[4]
- *Phase 1: Extraction.* To reduce the risk of poor healing, the 46 roots were extracted atraumatically by a specialist oral surgeon. The socket was packed and sutured and was monitored closely for healing.
- *Phase 2: Root canal treatment.* Root canal treatment was undertaken in the 31, 32, 33 and 43. Post spaces were left in the 33 and 43 to allow for post-retained magnetic root copings to retain the mandibular overdenture.

- *Phase 3: Composite resin restorations.* The 13, 21, 22 and 23 were built up with direct composite resin to aesthetic form. The roots of the 12 and 24 were domed over with composite resin.
- *Phase 4.* Jaw registration was completed in the retruded contact position (RCP) and the prosthetic envelope of movement was established for construction of upper and lower dentures.
- *Phase 5.* The mandibular teeth were prepared for cast root copings and these were bonded with resin cement (Panavia 21, Kurary Dental, USA) (Figures 4.22.4 and 4.22.5). These were provided due to the broken-down condition of the remaining teeth and to help retain the lower denture.
- *Phase 6.* The overdentures were assessed at try-in and magnets picked up in the mandibular complete denture. These were processed and delivered to yield the final result (Figure 4.22.6).
- Toothpaste with 5,000 ppm fluoride content (Duraphat® 5000 ppm Fluoride Toothpaste, Colgate-Palmolive, UK) was prescribed to reduce caries risk.
- A supportive maintenance regime was developed for the patient that included three-monthly visits to a dental hygienist for oral hygiene instruction and non-surgical periodontal treatment.[4]

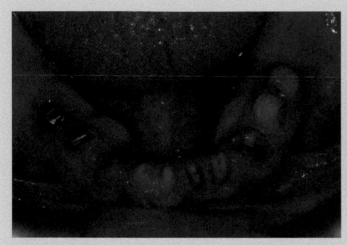

Figure 4.22.4 Roots prior to cementation of root copings.

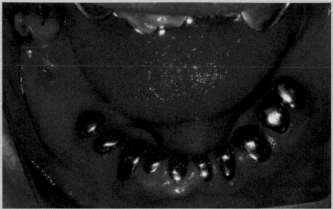

Figure 4.22.5 Post-operative mandibular view with root canal–treated teeth with cast copings.

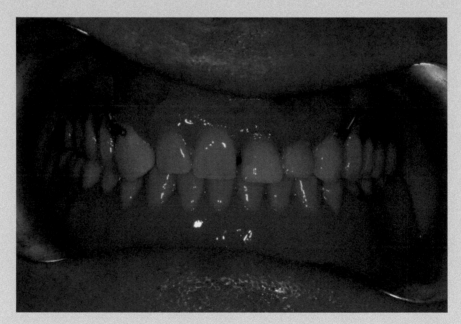

Figure 4.22.6 Post-operative view with final denture in situ.

Self-Study Questions

1. Following head and neck radiotherapy, which jaw is more likely to be at risk from ONJ?
   a. Equal risk
   b. Mandible
   c. Maxilla

2. When should newly diagnosed head and neck cancer patients be rendered dentally fit?
   a. Before radiotherapy
   b. During radiotherapy
   c. After radiotherapy

Answers are located at the end of the case

Self-Study Answers

1. b. Mandible[1]

2. a. Before radiotherapy[2]

References

1 Scottish Dental Clinical Effectiveness Programme (2017). *Oral Health Management of Patients at Risk of Medication-related Osteonecrosis of the Jaw*. NHS Education for Scotland, Edinburgh.

2 Moore C, McLister C, O'Neill C, et al. (2020). Pre-radiotherapy dental extractions in patients with head and neck cancer: a Delphi study. *Journal of Dentistry* 97: 103350.

3 Quilligan G, McKenna G, Allen PF (2016). The restorability assessment and endodontic access cavity interface. *Dental Update* 43: 933–938.

4 Moore C, McLister C, Cardwell C, et al. (2020). Dental caries following radiotherapy for head and neck cancer: a systematic review. *Oral Oncology* 100: 104484.

Case 23

Management of Primary Sjögren's Syndrome in a Partially Dentate Patient

With Contribution from Paul Brady

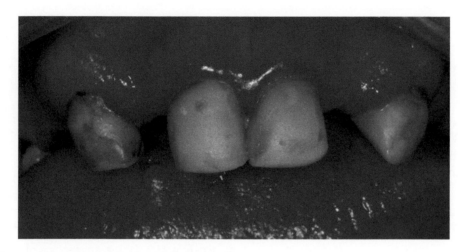

Figure 4.23.1 Patient's remaining upper teeth at initial presentation.

A. Case Story

A 68-year-old female was referred to a specialist in Oral Medicine. The referral letter stated that she was 'suffering from xerostomia for up to seven years. It is gradually getting worse and she now complains of a severely sore tongue and sore mucosa. She also suffers from rampant caries.' The patient was partially dentate in the upper arch and was considering implant-retained restorations to replace her missing teeth. Her remaining teeth were all heavily restored and there was evidence of extensive root caries (Figures 4.23.1 and 4.23.2). Her dental history over the past decade revealed a significant deterioration in her oral health, which included provision of multiple restorations and extractions. The patient had previously been diagnosed with primary Sjögren's syndrome, but was not receiving treatment at the time of referral.

LEARNING GOALS AND OBJECTIVES
- Appreciate that xerostomia and reduced salivary output are a common complaint in older patients[1]
- Understand the crucial role that saliva plays in preventing oral diseases such as caries; xerostomia and salivary hypofunction can have significant negative impacts on quality of life[2]
- Be aware that understanding the underlying aetiology of xerostomia is key to management; a number of systemic diseases can give rise to xerostomia, including Sjögren's syndrome, but other causes include polypharmacy and previous radiotherapy[3]

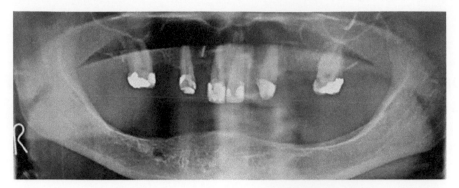

Figure 4.23.2 Radiographic assessment of patient.

B. Medical History

- Primary Sjögren's syndrome
- High blood pressure
- Arthritis affecting the fingers
- Previous treatment for breast cancer

C. Dental History

- History of dry mouth for many years
- Patient has lost many teeth due to caries
- Patient is now edentate in lower arch
- Struggling to adapt to removable prostheses in both upper and lower arches

D. Medications

- Propranolol hydrochloride (beta blocker) 80 mg twice per day
- Simvastatin (CoA reductase inhibitor) 40 mg once daily
- Aspirin (non-steroidal anti-inflammatory) 75 mg once daily

E. Social History

- Widowed
- Retired care assistant
- Living independently
- Previous smoker
- Does not consume alcohol

F. Extraoral Examination

- Temporomandibular joint (TMJ): nothing abnormal detected
- Muscles of mastication: nothing abnormal detected
- Lymph nodes: nothing abnormal detected

G. Soft Tissue Examination

- Red, erythematous mucosa in upper and lower arches
- Mucosa extremely dry (Figure 4.23.3)

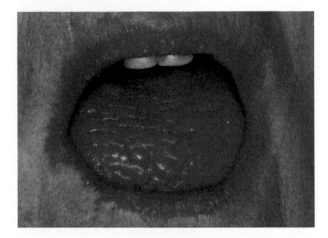

Figure 4.23.3 Clinical appearance of the patient's tongue.

H. Clinical Findings/Problem List

- Oral hygiene poor, plaque deposits present around gingival margins of remaining natural teeth
- Partially dentate in upper arch with six remaining carious teeth
- Remaining maxillary teeth very heavily restored
- Edentate in lower arch
- Mouth extremely dry
- Tooth charting:

		6		3		1	1		3		6		

- Basic periodontal examination:

–	3	–
–	–	–

I. Diagnoses

- Xerostomia secondary to Sjögren's syndrome
- Caries
- Partially dentate in maxilla and edentate in mandible

CLINICAL DECISION MAKING – DETERMINING FACTORS

- At the initial consultation the patient explained that she had difficulty talking and eating certain foods. She also mentioned that she had a stigma associated with her 'bad teeth'. There was nothing in her medical history of significance. At the initial consultation, she was swabbed for *Candida* and a blood sample was taken.
- As initial treatment the patient commenced on a Mycostatin suspension and dry mouth mouthwash gel and toothpaste (Biotene™, GlaxoSmithKline, USA).
- The blood test results showed a vitamin B12 deficiency and she was positive for *Candida*. The screening tests reported antibodies that were positive for primary biliary cirrhosis. She had a positive mitochondrial antibody test of 42.0 IU/mL (normal is 0–5). The incidental finding of tests consistent with primary biliary cirrhosis resulted in a referral to a hepatologist. She had been clinically asymptomatic for primary biliary cirrhosis.
- Oral involvement in Sjögren's syndrome gives rise to poor salivary flow, and difficulty speaking, swallowing and managing dentures. Accelerated dental caries is of particular dental importance.
- Primary Sjögren's syndrome occurs alone, whereas secondary Sjögren's syndrome occurs in association with other autoimmune diseases, frequently rheumatoid arthritis and systemic lupus erythematosus. Primary biliary cirrhosis is an autoimmune disease less commonly associated with Sjögren's syndrome.
- The patient continued to have a sore tongue and a very dry mouth. She was commenced on pilocarpine, which she found helped a lot with the dry mouth. She also developed dry eyes. It was recommended that she use salivary substitutes (Dry mouth oral gel, BioXtra, UK).
- The effects of xerostomia have had a profound impact on this woman's oral health. Rampant caries and in particular root caries have resulted in her having lost all her lower teeth and the remaining upper teeth are in poor condition.[2] The integrity of her oral mucosa has been affected. With the loss of teeth, she has also lost alveolar bone. The placement of implants is likely to help with the retention of her full lower denture; however, the prosthesis will need to be entirely implant borne, as her dry oral mucosa will not be able to accept any element of a tissue-borne prosthesis.[4] She is likely to require multiple implants to facilitate a properly functioning implant-retained full lower prosthesis.

Self-Study Questions

1. Compared to the healthy population, what is the prognosis for implants in Sjögren's syndrome cases?
   a. Better
   b. Comparable
   c. Worse

2. In cases of xerostomia, what can appropriate management include?
   a. Chlorhexidine mouthwash
   b. Citrus fruits
   c. Drinks based on citrus fruits
   d. Low pH sweets to stimulate salivary flow
   e. Water

3. What percentage of commonly prescribed medications list xerostomia as a potential side effect?
   a. 10%
   b. 25%
   c. 65%
   d. 80%

Answers are located at the end of the case

Self-Study Answers

1. b. Comparable[4]

2. e. Water[2]

3. d. 80%[2]

References

1 McKenna G, Burke FM (2010). Age-related oral changes. *Dental Update* 37: 519–523.

2 Turner MD, Ship JA (2007). Dry mouth and its effects on the oral health of elderly people. *Journal of the American Dental Association* 138: S15–S20.

3 Kossioni AE, Hajto-Bryk J, Janssens B, et al. (2018). Practical guidelines for physicians in promoting oral health in frail older adults. *Journal of the American Medical Directors Association* 19: 1039–1046.

4 Schimmel M, Srinivasan M, McKenna G, Müller F (2018). Effect of advanced age and/or systemic medical conditions on dental implant survival: a systematic review and meta-analysis. *Clinical Oral Implants Research* 29: 311–330.

Case 24

Management of Drug-Induced Gingival Overgrowth

With Contribution from Lewis Winning and Christopher Irwin

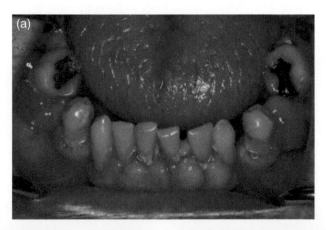

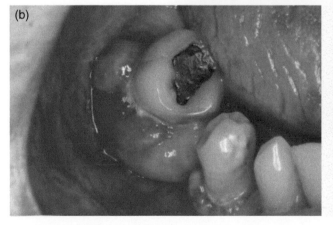

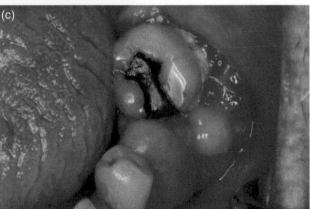

Figure 4.24.1 a–c Gingival overgrowth in the lower arch at initial presentation.

A. Case Story

A 73-year-old male was referred to the Periodontal Department of a dental school complaining of swollen gums. The patient's medical history included coronary hypertension, and his medication included amlodipine (10 mg once daily). He was previously a smoker, but had ceased 15 years previously. Clinical examination revealed moderate gingival overgrowth affecting the mandibular arch (Figure 4.24.1). Both buccal and lingual attached gingivae were affected. There was associated poor oral hygiene. Periodontal pocket probing revealed increased probing depths and generalised bleeding on probing.

LEARNING GOALS AND OBJECTIVES

- Recognise that several different drug categories have been reported to induce gingival overgrowth, with the most common being anticonvulsants, immunosuppressants and calcium channel blockers[1,2]
- Understand that these drugs appear to increase collagen synthesis and induce cellular changes in the host tissues; the incidence of gingival overgrowth is reported to be three times higher in males, as testosterone affects fibroblast proliferation and collagen stimulus
- Amlodipine is a calcium channel blocker commonly prescribed for the treatment of coronary hypertension and angina

B. Medical History

- Coronary hypertension controlled with medication
- High cholesterol

C. Dental History

- Irregular dental attender
- Attended general dental practitioner for the first time in two years when he noted swelling of his gums
- No previous history of periodontal disease

D. Medications

- Aspirin (non-steroidal anti-inflammatory) 150 mg daily
- Amlodipine (calcium channel blocker) 10 mg once daily
- Propranolol hydrochloride (beta blocker) 80 mg twice per day
- Simvastatin (CoA reductase inhibitor) 40 mg once daily

E. Social History

- Dairy farmer, still working
- Lives with wife and two sons
- Smokes approximately 5 cigarettes per day
- Alcohol: approximately 15 units per week

F. Extraoral Examination

- Temporomandibular joint (TMJ): nothing abnormal detected
- Muscle of mastication: nothing abnormal detected
- Lymph nodes: nothing abnormal detected

G. Soft Tissue Examination

- Moderate gingival overgrowth affecting the mandibular arch; both buccal and lingual attached gingivae were affected; periodontal pocket probing revealed increased probing depths and generalised bleeding on probing

H. Clinical Findings/Problem List

- Poor oral hygiene
- Partially dentate with some missing units
- Posterior missing units not replaced
- Gingival overgrowth affecting the mandibular arch
- Tooth charting:

	7	6		5	3	2	1	1	2	3	4		6		
	7		5		3	2	1	1	2	3		5		7	

- Basic periodontal examination:

1	1	1
3	3	3

I. Diagnosis

- Drug-induced gingival overgrowth (DIGO)

CLINICAL DECISION MAKING – DETERMINING FACTORS

- Amlodipine is a calcium channel blocker (CCB). CCBs are now the first-line drug of choice in the management of hypertension in patients >55 years.[3] Although this class of medication is generally well tolerated, CCBs have been recognised as a cause of DIGO. The reported prevalence of DIGO in patients taking CCBs varies widely, affecting between 5% and 80% of patients. The dihydropyridine group (amlodipine, nifedipine, felodipine) are the most commonly described CCBs involved in cases of DIGO. While the molecular mechanisms underlying the pathogenesis of drug-induced gingival enlargement are not fully understood, impaired collagen and extracellular matrix homeostasis, resulting in the accumulation of gingival connective tissues, is considered central to development of the condition.[4]

- Management options:
  - *Non-surgical periodontal therapy.* Plaque control should always be a first-line measure in an attempt to control the inflammatory component of DIGO. There is evidence that good oral hygiene and plaque removal decrease the degree of DIGO and improve periodontal health.[5]
  - *Surgical periodontal therapy.* Surgical treatment is only advocated where DIGO is severe, and should be combined with cause removal where possible and non-surgical management in the first instance.
  - *Consulting with patient's medical provider.* In recurrent or severe cases of DIGO, a patient's medical provider should be consulted regarding cessation of the causative medication and substitution with either another class or a cocktail of anti-hypertensive drugs. These include beta blockers, diuretics or ACE inhibitors. DIGO has not been reported with any of these drugs. A further option is substitution with another CCB that has a lower risk of inducing gingival enlargement (for example verapamil or isradipine). Multiple case reports have demonstrated the effectiveness of finding an alternative to the causative medication in DIGO.[6] Despite these options, physicians and patients are often reluctant to switch to other regimens, especially if the blood pressure is well controlled or other options have already been explored.

- In this instance non-surgical periodontal treatment was undertaken in combination with extensive oral hygiene instruction. After four appointments of non-surgical periodontal treatment, the gingival overgrowth had resolved considerably. The patient was discharged to his general dental practitioner, where he was placed on a regular maintenance schedule.

Self-Study Questions

1. Which of the following drugs cause gingival hyperplasia?
   a. Beta blockers
   b. Bronchodilators
   c. Calcium channel blockers
   d. Non-steroidal anti-inflammatories
   e. Proton pump inhibitors

2. What should be the first line of treatment for drug-induced gingival overgrowth?
   a. Antibiotic therapy
   b. Antimicrobial mouthwash
   c. Periodontal surgery
   d. Plaque control
   e. Subgingival scaling

Answers are located at the end of the case

Self-Study Answers

1. c. Calcium channel blockers

2. d. Plaque control

References

1 Seymour RA, Ellis JS, Thomason JM (2000). Risk factors for drug-induced gingival overgrowth. *Journal of Clinical Periodontology* 27: 217–223.
2 Mavrogiannis M, Ellis JS, Thomason JM, Seymour RA (2006). The management of drug-induced gingival overgrowth. *Journal of Clinical Periodontology* 33: 434–439.
3 Krause T, Lovibond K, Caulfield M, et al.; Guideline Development Group (2011). Management of hypertension: summary of NICE guidance. *British Medical Journal* 343: d4891.
4 Heasman PA, Hughes FJ (2014). Drugs, medications and periodontal disease. *British Dental Journal* 217: 411–419.
5 Castronovo G, Giuliana L, Fedon A, et al. (2014). The effect of nonsurgical periodontal treatment on the severity of drug-induced gingival overgrowth in transplant patients. *Quintessence International* 45: 115–124.
6 Khzam N, Bailey D, Yie HS, Makr MM (2016). Gingival enlargement induced by felodipine resolves with a conventional periodontal treatment and drug modification. *Case Reports in Dentistry* 2016: 1095927.

Case 25

Vital Bleaching to Improve the Aesthetics of Natural Teeth

With Contribution from Martina Hayes and Francis Burke

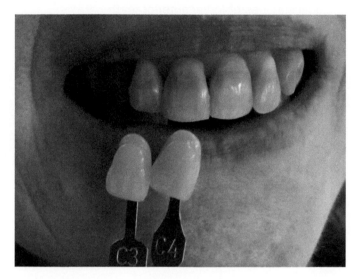

Figure 4.25.1 Patient at initial presentation; note the use of shade tabs in the initial photographs, which allows monitoring of tooth whitening.

A. Case Story

A 67-year-old female attended for a routine review. She was not having any discomfort from her teeth, but wanted to discuss with her dentist options to improve their aesthetics. Specifically, she wanted to have 'whiter teeth'. The patient was a longstanding regular attender and visited both the dentist and the hygienist every six months. In recent years she had noticed that her teeth had become darker in colour (Figure 4.25.1). She was not concerned about any other aspects of the aesthetics such as tooth position or size. The patient had researched tooth whitening and vital bleaching on the internet.

LEARNING GOALS AND OBJECTIVES

- Recognise that teeth do become darker as part of the normal physiological ageing process[1]; this is a combination of a number of factors, including thinning of the overlying enamel; gingival recession to reveal darker root surfaces; and staining
- Teeth whitening for vital teeth can be completed effectively, safely and with no operative interventions using up to 6% hydrogen peroxide products[2]
- Under European Union legislation (2011/84/EU), teeth whitening should be undertaken by a dentist and should always be accompanied by a comprehensive oral examination to identify and manage primary dental disease[3]; when providing tooth whitening for older patients, it is always advisable to remove underlying stains from the teeth prior to providing whitening products
- Patients should be made aware that some restorations may need to be changed after tooth whitening as they do not respond to the process

B. Medical History

- Hypertension
- High cholesterol
- Heartburn (gastric reflux), controlled with medication

C. Dental History

- Regular dental attender with very well-maintained dentition; patient attends dental hygienist for ultrasonic cleaning every six months
- Small number of missing posterior units, but not restored
- Composite resin restorations on upper anterior teeth, but well maintained
- Oral hygiene very good
- Patient drinks approximately four cups of black tea per day, which she feels has discoloured her teeth; patient also drinks red wine

D. Medications

- Simvastatin (CoA reductase inhibitor) 40 mg once daily
- Propranolol hydrochloride (beta blocker) 80 mg twice per day
- Omeprazole (proton pump inhibitor) 20 mg once daily

E. Social History

- Married with children at university
- Part-time shop assistant
- Non-smoker
- Alcohol use: eight units per week (red wine)

F. Extraoral Examination

- Temporomandibular joint (TMJ): asymptomatic click on left side opening

- Muscles of mastication: nothing abnormal detected
- Lymph nodes: nothing abnormal detected

G. Soft Tissue Examination

- No significant findings

H. Clinical Findings/Problem List

- Excellent oral hygiene
- Minimally restored dentition with some missing units
- No removable prostheses
- Small amount of supragingival calculus present on lingual surfaces of lower anterior teeth
- Shade of teeth at baseline: C4 (Vita Shade Guide)
- Tooth charting:

8	7	6		4	3	2	1	1	2	3	4	5	6	7	
	7		5	4	3	2	1	1	2	3	4	5	6		

- Basic periodontal examination:

1	1	1
1	2	1

I. Diagnosis

- Discoloured vital teeth in upper and lower arches

CLINICAL DECISION MAKING – DETERMINING FACTORS

- A detailed clinical examination revealed no evidence of primary dental disease.
- A simple treatment plan was developed with the patient to include ultrasonic scaling and polishing to remove staining on the teeth, followed by a course of vital tooth bleaching. More invasive forms of treatment such as provision of indirect restorations were not considered, as these are very destructive and therefore inappropriate in a case like this.
- At baseline the shade of the teeth was noted as C4 using a Vita Shade Guide (Figure 4.25.1). After cleaning, upper and lower impressions were taken in alginate (Hydrogum, Zhermack, Italy) using stock impression trays.
- Vacuum-formed bleaching trays were fabricated without reservoirs and provided to the patient.

- The patient was provided with a supply of 10% carbamide peroxide whitening gel (Polanight, SDI, Australia). She was also provided with detailed instructions on the use of the whitening gel as per the manufacturer's instructions:
  - Place a small amount of gel into each compartment of the bleaching tray.
  - Seat the tray, with the gel in place, around the teeth.
  - Wipe away any excess gel in the mouth or on the gums with a dry toothbrush.
  - Wear the bleaching trays for two hours per day or overnight.
  - After treatment remove the tray. Rinse the tray and mouth with lukewarm water.
  - Brush teeth.

- The patient was advised that tooth sensitivity is a recognised side effect of vital bleaching.[4] She was advised to use desensitising toothpaste in the bleaching tray overnight if she found that she was experiencing sensitivity.
- The patient returned for a review appointment four weeks after beginning tooth whitening. She was very pleased with the result, but it was decided to continue the treatment for a further four weeks to improve the shade further. The patient reported no sensitivity.

- At the conclusion of treatment, the patient's teeth were measured as shade C3 on the Vita Shade Guide (Figure 4.25.2).
- At six-month review the patient was still very happy with the aesthetics of her teeth and declined to have any composite restorations changed (Figure 4.25.3). She was advised that there may be some relapse over time, but that she could undertake a short top-up course of whitening if necessary using her existing trays for one week.

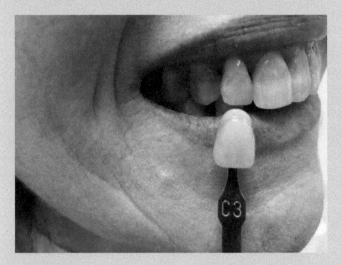

Figure 4.25.2 Patient's teeth recorded as shade C3 after a course of tooth whitening (shade tab included for reference).

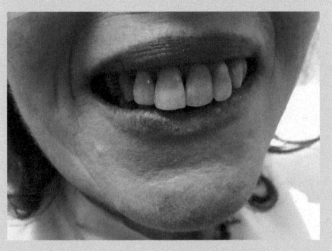

Figure 4.25.3 Final result six months after tooth whitening.

Self-Study Questions

1. What is the most common cause of tooth discoloration in older patients?
   a. The ageing process
   b. Coffee staining
   c. Red wine staining
   d. Smoking
   e. Tetracycline staining

2. You have a patient with dentine hypersensitivity. Which of the following topical agents would be least effective at relieving the patient's symptoms?
   a. Casein phosphopeptide–amorphous calcium phosphate (CPP-ACP) paste
   b. Carbamide peroxide gel

   c. Chlorhexidine thymol varnish
   d. Fluoride varnish
   e. Resin varnish

3. Which of the following conditions is not amenable to bleaching with hydrogen peroxide?
   a. Ageing
   b. Amelogenesis imperfecta
   c. Fluorosis
   d. Pulpal haemorrhagic products
   e. Tobacco staining

Answers are located at the end of the case

Self-Study Answers

1. a. The ageing process[1]

2. b. Carbamide peroxide gel

3. b. Amelogenesis imperfecta

References

1 McKenna G, Burke FM (2010). Age-related oral changes. *Dental Update* 37: 519–523.

2 Kelleher MGD, Djemal S, Al-Khayatt AS, et al. (2017). Bleaching and bonding for the older patient. *Dental Update* 38: 298–303.

3 EU Council Directive 2001/84/EU (2011). *European Union*, Brussels.

4 Kothari S, Gray AR, Lyons K, et al. (2019). Vital bleaching and oral health-related quality of life in adults: a systematic review. *Journal of Dentistry* 84: 22–29.

INDEX

Page locators in **bold** indicate tables. Page locators in *italics* indicate figures. This index uses letter-by-letter alphabetization.

Clinical Cases in Gerodontology, First Edition. Edited by Gerry McKenna, Finbarr Allen, and Francis Burke.
© 2021 John Wiley & Sons Ltd. Published 2021 by John Wiley & Sons Ltd.